INSIDE TAI CHI

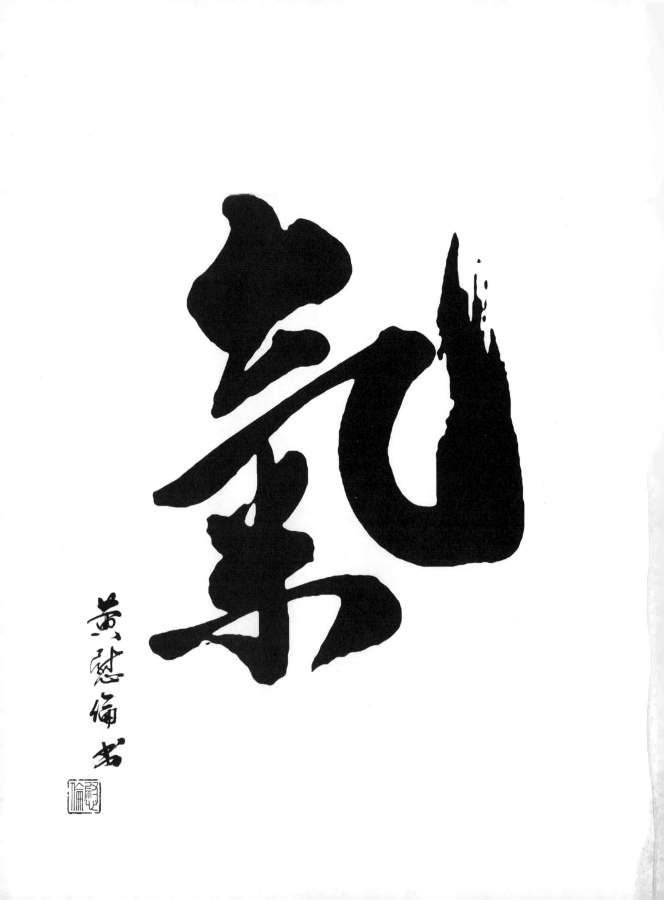

INSIDE TAI CHI

Hints, Tips, Training, & Process for Students and Teachers

JOHN LOUPOS

YMAA Publication Center
Boston, Mass. USA

YMAA Publication Center
Main Office
4354 Washington Street
Boston, Massachusetts, 02131
1-800-669-8892 • www.ymaa.com • ymaa@aol.com

10   9   8   7   6   5   4   3   2   1

Editor: Lynn Teale
Cover Calligraphy: Master Wei Lun Huang
Drawings: Vasiliki Belezos
Cover Design: Katya Popova
Anatomical images from LifeART, SuperAnatomy, Copyright ©1994, Lippincott Williams
& Wilkins, a Wolters Kluwer Company.

Publisher's Cataloging in Publication
(Prepared by Quality Books Inc.)

Loupos, John, 1953-
    Inside tai chi : hints, tips, training & process for
students nad teachers / John Loupos.—1st ed.
        p. cm.
        Includes index.
        LCCN: 2002101834
        ISBN: 1-886969-10-8

    1. Tai chi.   I. Title.

GV504.L68 2002   613.7'148
                                QBI02-200221

Disclaimer:
    The author and publisher of this material are NOT RESPONSIBLE in any
manner whatsoever for any injury which may occur through reading or following
the instructions in this manual.
    The activities, physical or otherwise, described in this material may be too
strenuous or dangerous for some people, and the reader(s) should consult a physician before engaging in them.

Printed in Canada

Contents

PART ONE: BASIC THEORY AND INTRA-PERSONAL PRACTICE SKILLS

Chapter 1. Introduction 3

Chapter 2. Ch'i, Where Life Begins 9

Chapter 3. Understanding Stress as It Relates to T'ai Chi 19

Chapter 4. The Importance of Rooting, How to Get Yours and Keep It 33

Foreword

This book is an important contribution to the body of writings on the art of T'ai Chi Ch'uan. Rather than just another methodological or philosophical approach, it seeks to answer a much more fundamental question; namely, how can the study of this ancient system of mind/body practice actually help me live my life more deeply, heartfully and well? Beyond the health and potential self-defense benefits typically described in both classic and modern T'ai Chi treatises, what possible contribution can the study of T'ai Chi make to my personal and spiritual development?

In contrast to some other better known and highly popularized martial art styles which, at least in the West, usually emphasize highly macho, aggressive, and violent images, T'ai Chi is best known for it's positive effects on health and longevity. As a result, its classic quality as an effective and elegant system of self-defense is often overlooked. While this may dismay some orthodox martially inclined practitioners, many more gifted teachers and students of the art, including some highly accomplished martial artists, have welcomed the growth of T'ai Chi. Its well-deserved reputation as a system for promoting health has widened its appeal and brought numerous benefits to many more people.

As public interest in all types of Oriental mind/body disciplines continues to grow, there has also been the beginning of an understanding that the training of attention, awareness of bodily energy, and stillness-in-action, fostered by this art are an integral part of its tradition and highest expression. The fact that the cultivation of attention is also the foundation of all authentic spiritual practices places the correct practice of T'ai Chi at the doorstep of spiritual work. Ultimately, any spiritual practice should help the practitioner live with greater intelligence, compassion and the ability to remain in the present moment whether one lives in the midst of ordinary life or in a monastery. The correct practice of T'ai Chi holds this promise for the dedicated student.

The possibility that T'ai Chi can actively support one's inner psychological and spiritual growth makes this question particularly relevant and timely to those of you who are just beginning this journey of discovery of this art. But it is equally important for those of us who for many years have been committed practitioners. Anyone involved seriously in the study and practice of the art—beginning students, long term practitioners and teachers—may at some point ask themselves what deeper psychological and spiritual benefits they may have gained from many months or years of investment of their time and energy in their practice. For example, do I experience myself as more vital, centered, calm and aware in my dealings with people and events in my life? Am I freer in my emotional responses to stress and conflict in my life? Have I become a person of greater integrity and depth as a result of my dedicated study of T'ai Chi? The answer to these questions may reveal a great deal about the nature of a student's core motivation for studying T'ai Chi as well as the intent and quality of the teaching they have received.

As someone who for many years has been graced to study with a number of eminent and extraordinary T'ai Chi Ch'uan lineage holders, I have periodically asked myself these same questions. To a certain extent, I feel that my work on the deeper aspects of the art of T'ai Chi has supported the development and emergence of presence, harmony and spirit in my daily life. These specific qualities, especially the cultivation of a consistent moment-to-moment bodily awareness of Ch'i (Qi) or life force in both stillness and activity are extremely important in my own development. That this process has been aided and abetted by my personal practice of the Gurdjieff Work, Buddhist sitting meditation, and Qigong, does not diminish the importance of T'ai Chi in shaping my ability to respond gracefully and with spontaneous intelligence to the challenges of life.

To date, exploration of the deeper psychological and spiritual implications of the study of T'ai Chi have not received much professional attention. A few practitioner-writers have occasionally speculated about aspects of T'ai Chi that reflects elements of Taoist spirituality such as Yin/Yang and the Five Element theories. However, to the best of my knowledge, with one or two exceptions, notably, Peter Ralston's pioneering early work, *Integrity of Being*, few writers have attempted to investigate both practically and systematically the broader question of how T'ai Chi affects one's inner life and mind/body unity.

Inside Tai Chi—Hints, Tips, Training, & Process for Students & Teachers addresses this challenge ably and well. John Loupos has taken up this task honestly, humbly and boldly. He writes directly from his many years of dedicated study and teaching of T'ai Chi as well as an excellent grounding in general principles of integrative mind/body medicine and related systems of self-development, including Oriental medicine and Taoism. Since John is a T'ai Chi brother and friend of mine for over twenty years, I know something about his willingness and ability to venture into unexplored territory such as this, and effectively communicate his discoveries to others in ways that are helpful to both beginners and advanced practitioners.

However, ultimately, you dear reader will make this determination yourself. If, as a beginner, you decide to commit yourself to the study of T'ai Chi; or, as an advanced practitioner or teacher, wish to explore the psychological and spiritual benefits of this art for yourself and your students, you will find many valuable ideas and insights in this book. In any case, *Inside Tai Chi—Hints, Tips, Training, & Process for Students & Teachers* will give you a very helpful perspective for this inquiry, as well as a number of specific tools to assist you along the way in your personal discovery of the deeper aspects and benefits of the "Grand Ultimate"—T'ai Chi Ch'uan.

Many blessings to you on your journey.
Gunther M. Weil, Ph.D.

Preface

"What a long strange trip it's been"
—Jerry Garcia & The Grateful Dead

I want to begin here by sharing a bit of my own journey, and in so doing set a tone for the underlying theme of this book, which is one of personal process via the study of T'ai Chi.

The decisions we each make on a daily basis, as well as the external manifestations of our various experiences, are certainly important. All too often we live out our day-to-day existences caught up in what is going on around us. We fail to indulge ourselves the time, or neglect to make the effort, to really notice what is happening inside us, below the surface. Paying attention to, or noticing, our own personal (or more accurately, intra-personal) process, is a dynamic process in and of itself. Such intrapersonal awareness can reveal the reasons and motivating factors behind our thoughts and behaviors in order to help us discern their truer meaning; as well as the impact they have on us in our daily lives. When we are more attuned to our own intra-personal processes our lives become more fully our own. Towards the realization of this process, T'ai Chi can be an effective tool.

I have written this book in the hope that what I have to share will in some way enrich your own T'ai Chi process. If you are already involved in an ongoing study, or if you are considering T'ai Chi as a resource for yourself, this book may inspire you directly onwards. I also hope to inspire you a bit more indirectly by reaching out and sharing some of my own personal experiences. This sharing can help validate the occasional step backwards, miscue, or disillusionment that you are sure to encounter sooner or later as a T'ai Chi practitioner. Experiences of "failure," or setback, can be enormously valuable learning tools, provided the experience is not wasted. In fact, as failure can provide the opportunity for a unique kind of learning, such setbacks can be every bit as valuable to you and your T'ai Chi as the more commonly sought after technical proficiency. It bears repeating that the only experiences that are truly wasted are those that we regard as such.

My own martial journey dates back to 1966, when living in suburbia at age 13, I took up the study of Karate. Originally, I was drawn to the martial arts due to their reputed mystical qualities. Even at that point in my life I was more of a seeker then a fighter, although I recall that I did have something of a problem at the time with local bullies. As luck would have it, I fell in with a teacher who had some modicum of spirituality. It was not long at all before I found myself taken with him and hanging on his every word. Consequently, I was shaken when, without notice, he disappeared when I was just two years into my studies. I later learned that he had left his wife and run off with one of the women in his class. And so, here was my first disillusionment. I never saw this teacher again, but I still hold him in my heart.

When my teacher left, his top student assumed leadership of the school, and so I was able to continue my studies. After several months this teacher left for what was supposed to be a temporary professional assignment. I never saw him again either. I was next in the pecking order, and though just fifteen years old at the time, I was asked by our headquarters to manage the school and to conduct classes on an interim basis as another adult teacher was due to relocate to the area shortly. "Shortly" turned into six months and the first thing my new mentor did on his eventual arrival was announce that he could only teach on Saturdays due to the demands of work and school. So the fuller burden of running the school remained squarely on my shoulders. Except for a two-year hiatus during which I grew my hair long and hitchhiked around the country, I spent the next five or six years practicing and teaching Karate.

By the time I had reached the seven-year mark, Karate had begun to feel limited to me in the rewards it offered, but it was still the best (only) game in town. That was, until a friend took me to see a Kung Fu demonstration in 1973. I was awe struck; it was love at first sight. In comparison with the linear, militaristic moves I had been practicing during my years of Karate, the graceful fluidity of Kung Fu captured and held my attention.

Shortly after this first exposure, I undertook the study of Kung Fu, (initially the Bak Sil Lum, or Northern Shaolin, style and later, the Bak Sing Choy Lay Fut style), commuting daily, sometimes twice, to Boston's Chinatown from my home some thirty miles away. (Fortunately, this was before parking tickets were computerized.) My new Sifu took me under his wing, and seemed to appreciate me all the more for my preexisting studies and my organized (thank you, Karate) teaching style. In less than a year's time, he had me teaching classes and working full time at his school.

As part of my overall studies he taught me my first T'ai Chi form (just the moves, mind you) and almost immediately encouraged me to go forth and teach it to others. Having no reason to believe otherwise, I thought I knew T'ai Chi. Ignorance can indeed be blissful.

Eventually, this first Sifu of mine heeded bad advice from other students and opened up too many schools too fast. He spread himself too thin and ended up losing everything. Around this same time, I had a failed romance with a student who, coincidentally, was quite wealthy. Purportedly angry with me for failing to marry my student girlfriend, my Sifu estranged himself from me, and soon left town. Only later did I learn that he had been writing to a fellow Sifu that he had a student (me) who was going to marry a rich girl and support him for the rest of his life. So much for altruism.

After our geographical parting of the ways I opened my own school, and still hungering for more knowledge, took up studies with another master (the same master, as it turned out, in whom my first Sifu had been confiding). Right up front, this master disclosed to me the content of my first Sifu's correspondences, assuring me that the politics of my previous situation would have no bearing on my future studies in his school. However, when I explained to my new Sifu that I sought a spiritual path along with my external training, he made it clear that he had no interest whatsoever in any of that. This Sifu only practiced Kung Fu and snickered openly at T'ai Chi. So I was surprised when one day, after his return from a trip to China, he suddenly began teaching T'ai Chi. Still anxious to learn whatever I could, and remain properly respectful, I jumped on board. His form was similar to, yet different from, the one I had learned earlier. This newer version of the T'ai Chi form seemed to emphasize lower stances. Now my T'ai Chi was even better than before, or so I thought.

Several years after undertaking my studies with this second Sifu, I had occasion to meet a teacher of the Tao who taught alchemical energy meditation and Ch'i Kung practices. I finally had the opportunity I had been waiting for to add some spiritual component to my practice. However, my studies with this Tao master presented a problem for my Kung Fu Sifu who felt stung by what he perceived as my divided loyalties. Try as I might, I could not convince him that my spiritual/internal practices posed no threat to our relationship. But he was adamant, and made such a big deal of this issue that it put an irreparable strain on our relationship. Eventually, the rigidity of his beliefs allowed him to realize his own worst fears about me, and we parted badly.

Meanwhile, everything was copacetic with my Tao master, until he started to gain wide recognition and an international following. More recognition meant more students, more teaching, more traveling, books, cassettes, videos, posters, flash cards, and more rules to ensure the conformity and compliance of his followers. Believe me, this took enormous sums of money and equally great concentrations of time and effort to raise that money. Eventually, this teacher left for greener pastures, and I was left to wonder, after going through five teachers in twenty-five years, what my role was in this pattern.

At some point I had come to realize that Sifus and Masters are all just human, and not necessarily any more evolved than the rest of us seekers. I made the determination at this time to avoid future complications by not getting entangled in any further teacher/student relationships, at least not with me as the student. Yet I hungered to learn more. Notwithstanding my earlier experiences and my decision to eschew masters, I decided to try hosting another teacher, whom I had met some years earlier, for a workshop at my school. (Not questing for another Sifu, after all I had been through, did not mean that I was through learning what others had to teach.)

Wei Lun Huang was a renowned T'ai Chi master who had married a Kung Fu teaching colleague of mine. Exercising caution to avoid any repetition of my earlier experiences, I had observed Master Huang from a close, but safe, distance for several years. I wanted a pretty clear sense of who he was and of what he really did before committing myself through any direct contact. When I finally did bring Master Huang to teach a seminar at my school the experience was rewarding, if not humbling, to say the least. Master Huang brought none of the pretensions of my earlier teachers and seemed to me genuine in every regard. Despite the reservations I had felt about following another Sifu, I found myself charmed and disarmed by Wei Lun Huang's demeanor. His humility, compassion, and genuine tolerance for the individuality of other persons, was rivaled only by his mastery of internal arts. Here at last was a master of such a caliber that he did not need to control others in order to validate his own mastery. As my guard gradually lowered, this new found relationship took root and I came finally to accept Master Wei Lun Huang as my Sifu and as my friend.

Now, as I look back over my years in martial arts, I realize I have had many challenges along my path. Perhaps the greatest challenge of all has been knowing what it was that I sought, and then recognizing it when I finally found it. There were many occasions when I thought I held my grail in the palm of my hand, only to find that I was holding just another illusion or transitional experience. I am truly fortunate in not having been irreparably soured by my many missteps. Had I been more goal oriented and less process oriented, it is possible that I might have left martial arts in pursuit of a different path entirely. As it is, I am thankful for good times and bad. Not a day goes by that I do not count my blessings, both in terms of what I have learned and in terms of the prospects I have for adding further to my knowledge. I believe that the key for me has been my persistence and the firmly held conviction that I can accomplish whatever I set my mind to. That belief, along with my willingness and ability to observe my own process nonjudgmentally so as to cull life's lessons from wherever they are to be had, is what kept me on my path and brought me to where I am today. Now it is my intent to share some of what I have learned in hopes that it may be of benefit to you.

Thank you for this opportunity.
Sifu John Loupos

Prelude

Note: I use the terms T'ai Chi and T'ai Chi Ch'uan casually and interchangeably throughout this book.

Let me begin by assuring the reader that even though I have been practicing T'ai Chi since 1974, it is only with caution and the most respectful of intentions that I present myself as a spokesperson for any T'ai Chi community other than my own. There are a great many players/teachers who are more skilled and who have been involved in T'ai Chi for longer than I, and I remain humbly cognizant of the fact that my own learning remains an ongoing process.

In writing this book, I strove to bridge the gap between three different worlds. One world is the existing T'ai Chi community comprised of individuals who are typically understated but self-assured, as well as practical and discriminating. A second world is comprised of those untold numbers of individuals who have yet to experience T'ai Chi as a next step in their own personal journey. In regard to this group, I hope to present T'ai Chi Ch'uan as an exciting and viable resource for better living on many levels. A third group includes all those who make their way as health care service providers such as psychotherapists, bodyworkers, chiropractors, acupuncturists, et al, and an increasing number of western medical professionals, especially those physicians and nurses, who may be oriented towards minimally invasive healing modalities. I bear this group in mind because I feel strongly that T'ai Chi is a complementary, but underutilized, resource that can be gainfully explored as an adjunctive natural healing therapy. Hopefully, this book will cast new and valuable light on the subject of T'ai Chi for each of these three groups.

Many fine volumes on T'ai Chi already exist. However, a goodly number of those books currently available are scholarly in their approach, or written with a fairly narrow scope, i.e., this style or aspect of T'ai Chi or that. Consequently, they find their greatest concentration of appreciative readers within the already existing T'ai Chi community. While other books do a splendid technical job explaining the classical principles and postures of T'ai Chi, this book is written more from a perspective of mind/body philosophy and psychology rather than as just another "How to Do the Form" guide. I have included some useful "How to" technical tips in order to give readers valuable hands-on guidance to improve their Tai Chi practice. My orientation however, is more one of Tai Chi as an "intrapersonal process" rather than Tai Chi as merely another exercise or martial art system. This book represents a compendium of my own learning experiences along with information and guidance on how you can improve the effects of your own practice on your life overall, or enhance your skills if you are a teacher. Newer T'ai Chi students should bear in mind that many of the skills described herein can only be achieved over time and as a result of extensive practice, practice that is ideally correct in its attempt to adhere to the principles.

My hope is that this book will serve as some small catalyst in the T'ai Chi growth experience for all those who read it, students and teachers alike. Despite the technical divergences between different styles, I believe that embodied within this text are thoughts, ideas, and perspectives that may well have something to offer even the more experienced practitioners in their understanding of T'ai Chi and/or how it can be more effectively taught.

Disclaimer

Though the exercises contained in this book are generally non-jarring and quite safe, prudence would dictate that you consult with your physician or health care provider prior to embarking on any new exercise program.

Romanization of Chinese Words

This book uses the Wade-Giles romanization system of Chinese to English. There are two other systems currently in use. These are the Pinyin and the Yale systems. The cover of this book presents the Wade-Giles romanization without apostrophes in order to simplify cataloging

Some common conversions:

Wade-Giles	Pinyin	Pronunciation
Ch'i	Qi	chē
Ch'i Kung	Qigong	chē kŭng
Chin Na	Qin Na	chĭn nă
Kung Fu	Gongfu	gŏng foo
T'ai Chi Ch'uan	Taijiquan	tī jē chüén

For more information, please refer to *The People's Republic of China: Administrative Atlas*, *The Reform of the Chinese Written Language*, or a contemporary manual of style.

How to Use This Book

How We Learn New Things. There are several approaches to learning something new. Either one of the first two of these can be employed when you have no previous knowledge of a given subject. The first of these approaches is vicarious learning, or learning about something indirectly as a result of reading, being taught, or observing what others know or have themselves been taught. Vicarious learning gives us the opportunity to experience a whole world of knowledge that we would not likely encounter or absorb otherwise such as ancient history, or ideas and philosophies of diverse cultures and great minds. Vicarious learning is what we undergo primarily as young students in school, and is an efficient way for us to learn for ourselves what has already been learned by others without needing to start all over from scratch.

A second approach to learning is that which results from direct experience. Direct learning stems from direct personal experience, and in many cases may be subject to our own subjective interpretation. For example, you can be told that it takes ten minutes to walk around the block (i.e. a distance of one mile). Knowing that information vicariously, and knowing it because you have walked around the block are two different kinds of knowledge, even if the facts of the matter remain the same. For one person, walking around the block may seem pleasantly long, for someone else the same walk may feel disappointingly short. Direct learning usually entails some aspect of personal discovery. Another example might be that you know in your mind that exercise such as T'ai Chi is good for you, but you will not derive the benefits of such knowing until you get moving and actually integrate a regular practice routine into your life. Both these kinds of learning, vicarious and direct, are useful and unique in what they have to offer.

A third kind of learning is hybrid learning. Hybrid learning is vicarious learning that is based on direct knowledge already held by you. It is a way of acquiring a different slant, or perspective, on something you have already had direct experience with but does not entail the acquisition of brand new knowledge per se. With hybrid learning, you can use new vicarious information to augment existing knowledge. If for example, someone were to tell you of a convenient shortcut for a route with which you were already directly familiar, you probably would not need to go out and actually try the short cut to know that it works. Instead, you might say, "Aha, this will save me time," linking the new information immediately to that already held. The more you already know about something, the more useful and efficient hybrid learning is because of the way it piggybacks on old knowledge.

What This Means for You. Any or all of these approaches to learning may be called into play as you read this book, assimilating the knowledge contained herein. Which approach works best for you will depend on whatever previous experience you may already have, as well as your commitment to learning (about) T'ai Chi.

In addition to providing a theoretical basis for the study of T'ai Chi, this book will guide you in simple ways to experiment practically with T'ai Chi's most fundamental principles:

1. Relaxing your breath
2. Relinquishing stress
3. Feeling your earth-root
4. Improving your posture

Experimenting with these T'ai Chi principles will help you enjoy the benefits of direct experience.

If you are a novice, this book will help you to learn, vicariously, a great deal about this ancient art so that you will be in a position to make a well informed decision as to whether, and how, to proceed with any actual study of T'ai Chi.

For those readers with limited T'ai Chi experience (one to five years), there may be somewhat less novelty in the theory but plenty of opportunity for new knowledge to be gained via the guided exercises. Also, many of the practice hints and training tips contained herein will undoubtedly prove helpful in improving your current practice.

For more experienced practitioners and T'ai Chi teachers, there will be incrementally less vicarious information, but tremendous opportunity for hybrid learning.

For ease of readership, in deference to the T'ai Chi novice reader, this book has been divided into three sections. The chapters of the first section do contain some exercises geared towards direct experience, but mostly address T'ai Chi's theoretical and practical application as an intra-personal development tool.

Practical technical information will be found later in those chapters comprising the second section.

The third, and final, section contains reference appendices, personal accounts, and lecture transcripts along with some personal musings.

Happy reading!

Acknowledgments

I have worked with many fine external and internal teachers over the years since I began my martial arts training in 1966. First thanks go to my first teacher, the late Sensei Howard Flynn, who guided me as a young Karate student in my initial attempts at martial proficiency and personal development.

I thank Henry Thom, a subsequent mentor, for introducing me to my first Sifu, Chin Bing Cheung, under whom I studied Bak Sil Lum, Bak Sing Choy Lay Fut, and Yang style T'ai Chi.

I spent many years learning Praying Mantis Kung Fu with Grandmaster Chan Pui.

Also, I have warm memories of the late Choy Lay Fut Grandmaster, Lee Koon Hung for being my friend and sharing generously of his knowledge.

I thank Dr. Gunther Weil for starting me on the path of the Tao, eventually to study with his teacher, Master Mantak Chia, who furthered my T'ai Chi education and taught me Taoist meditation and Ch'i Kung disciplines. Special thanks also to Dr. Weil for his foreword.

My thanks as well go to Dr. Xie Pe Qui of Beijing who shared so openly of his Yin style Ba Gua and healing methods.

Finally, and most enthusiastically, I wish to extend my appreciation to my friend and teacher, Master Wei Lun Huang. Master Huang redefined my world by teaching me his Yang style T'ai Chi, Classical Ba Gua, and Liu He Ba Fa, and by setting such a fine example of how to actually *live* one's T'ai Chi.

I wish to add my gratitude as well for my many students over the years, who have unknowingly guided me, inspiring me through their own efforts to learn, ever serving as mirrors for myself as a practitioner, as a teacher, and as a human being.

I also want to extend my thanks to certain individuals whose help in completing this book has been of immeasurable value: Lynn Teale, my editor at YMAA; Gretchen Sassone for her limitless generosity in providing thoughtful and provocative editorial advice, and my illustrator, Vasiliki Belezos for her outstanding artwork. As an intuitive artist, Vicki uses stillness and motion to reveal the essence of refracted imagery. Her illustrations effectively capture my ideas and will allow readers easy visual access to my message.

I also thank Diana Frost, a T'ai Chi teaching colleague, for her help in clarifying concepts in the "how to" sections and elsewhere throughout this text.

My thanks go as well to Dr. Ron Milestone, and to my student Bob Doyle, for taking time out of their busy schedules to proof the text and provide editorial feedback. Thanks also to my many friends and colleagues who proffered their advice in one way or another at my behest.

Finally, I want to thank my son, Chris, who has been all any father could ask for, and who inadvertently provided me the incentive to undertake the joyful task of writing in the first place.

BASIC T'AI CHI THEORY AND INTRA-PERSONAL PRACTICE SKILLS

CHAPTER 1

Introduction

A Brief History of T'ai Chi Ch'uan

The slow motion art of T'ai Chi is said by some to have been first developed by Chang San-feng during the Song dynasty (A.D. 960–1278). According to legend, as a young man Chang was scholarly and well-traveled. He studied martial arts extensively during his travels, and spent ten years training at Shaolin where he reputedly mastered all their exercises. In his later years he is said to have studied Taoist alchemy.

The exact origin of T'ai Chi Ch'uan is uncertain. One story says Chang created T'ai Chi as the result of a dream he had. Another story had Chang observing a conflict between a bird and a snake, alleging his observations served as a basis for T'ai Chi. In either case T'ai Chi certainly exemplifies principles drawn from the Taoist tradition and from the *I-Ching* (See Glossary). Quite a number of excellent books are available today detailing the origins and historical philosophy of T'ai Chi. The curious reader is referred to those many volumes currently available for more detailed information.

Since Chang's day there have evolved several different styles of T'ai Chi Ch'uan. Aside from those factors that distinguish the different styles it is true as well that individual teachers often have their own individual approaches. Though the different systems vary in ways that lend each its particular identity there are also denominators common to each. The following is a primer to familiarize the reader with the most common and beneficial aspects of traditional T'ai Chi Ch'uan.

A T'ai Chi Primer: T'ai Chi Ch'uan Explained

The T'ai Chi Classics say...

> *"T'ai Chi can make you Solid as a Mountain,*
> *Supple as a Willow, and Fluid as a Great River."*

In today's high tech world even the most basic of our needs have become conspicuously dependent on technological gadgets of one sort or another. Activities as simple as walking or running call for special shoes, pulse monitors, or treadmills (even the lower end models being fully computerized for maximum convenience). In refreshing contrast to this state of affairs we are gifted with the ancient art of T'ai Chi Ch'uan. No designer lycra outfits, no digital thingys, no rackets, bells, or whistles...T'ai Chi is decidedly low tech.

T'ai Chi Ch'uan is the most widely practiced martial art/health care system in the world today. In China, millions of people commit to beginning each day with its practice. This is due largely to the fact that T'ai Chi is understood to offer those who practice it a range of benefits for mind, body and soul.

At this time, as we embark on a new millennium, T'ai Chi has become firmly rooted in our own western culture as well. Only recently have organized studies begun to explore the reputed health benefits of T'ai Chi. Yet, centuries of empirical evidence lay claim to T'ai Chi's efficacy as a health care and wellness modality. In China, T'ai Chi has typically been indicated for a wide range of chronic illnesses, including, but not limited to:

1. Back or knee problems
2. Hypertension and other stress related issues
3. Circulatory system disorders
4. Nervous system disorders
5. Addictions
6. Arthritis
7. Asthma
8. Mental illness

Tai Chi's application in addressing medical issues such as these remains largely untapped here in the west. Nevertheless, there is little question that T'ai Chi has a great deal to offer, and if the growing number of medical studies citing T'ai Chi for its wide-ranging benefits are any indication of this, then western science and medicine are starting to sit up and take notice.

Today almost everyone has had some exposure to T'ai Chi via the various media. Film clips or documentaries on China often depict (albeit briefly) groups of people practicing early morning T'ai Chi exercises. In China, the parks and waterfronts are full of people who begin each day with this healthy slow-motion routine. The Chinese regard T'ai Chi as an official exercise and as a national treasure. The effective manner in which it contributes to their vast population's wellness and reputed vitality is so important for a country historically lacking in sophisticated medical resources.

T'ai Chi made its first great leap forward into the American stream of consciousness back in 1993, with Bill Moyers' critically acclaimed PBS series "*Healing and the Mind.*" Since that time, T'ai Chi's growth in America has been exponential. Yet, a clear understanding of the purpose and intricacies of this ancient art remains elusive, even for teachers experienced in other fields of martial arts, let alone for the average layperson. T'ai Chi is like the proverbial iceberg in that there is more to it than meets the eye.

By way of explanation, "T'ai Chi Ch'uan" is a generic term. There are several different styles of T'ai Chi popularly practiced. Common to each of the different T'ai Chi systems is a slow motion movement routine. Beyond that the differences depend on the teacher with whom you speak. But one thing that T'ai Chi emphatically is not is slowed down Karate or Kung Fu. The principles of genuine T'ai Chi differ fundamentally from those of harder style martial arts. T'ai Chi as a martial art maintains its own autonomy.

Although T'ai Chi's benefits are wide-ranging and not limited to those listed below, I understand its practice to be of particular value in four regards:

1. The cultivation of Ch'i, or life force energy
2. Exercising and conditioning the body on a very deep level
3. Learning to understand and apply the inner structure of the body
4. Learning to be focused in the moment.

These four areas are pretty much all encompassing. Any of T'ai Chi's other benefits can arguably be assigned to one of these categories. Some of these ideas may seem a bit foreign and difficult to grasp at first, but concealed within these concepts is the magic that T'ai Chi has to offer. It is however, the actual living of these principles that enables the T'ai Chi practitioner to experience renewed health and well-being on all levels. T'ai Chi students may also experience the feeling of being more integrated both with themselves and with their environment. It is the living of these principles that serves as the focal point for this book. [A fifth and separate equally important regard that begs mention, but which I will not address in detail in this book, is T'ai Chi's application as a fighting art.]

Life Force Energy, or Ch'i, is what animates humans as individual living beings. T'ai Chi Ch'uan exerts a gentle balance on one's life force (Ch'i) energy, and promotes improved health and longevity, and an enhanced quality of life. Cultivating a practical understanding and reservoir of Ch'i for self-healing or for martial arts purposes entails a very specialized approach that is best learned from others, who are already knowledgeable in such practice.

T'ai Chi body conditioning is unique in how it simultaneously challenges and addresses the needs of body and mind. Slow, gentle, and continuous, T'ai Chi stretching increases the body's range of motion while improving muscle and soft tissue tone and resilience. This manifests on a level deep enough to begin to counter the long-term effects of chronic stress/tension/pain that many people carry. After just a few months of practice, T'ai Chi students often find themselves able to enjoy activities and a freedom of movement thought long lost.

The *inner structure* of T'ai Chi refers to the anatomically correct alignment of the skeletal frame and connective tissues. Advanced level T'ai Chi is quite precise and entails an exact, often frustratingly subtle, positioning of the body's various components. The bones, tendons, and ligaments must be aligned "just so" in order to facilitate a mechanical advantage in movement or stillness. This can take

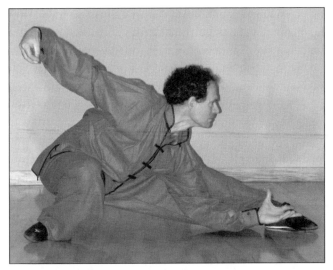

Figure 1-1. Snake Creeps Down

quite some time to master, but once grasped the benefits of improved posture, rooting, and economy of motion become self-evident.

Finally, we are *learning to be in the moment*. As simple as this sounds it is probably the concept most challenging for the average westerner to actually implement. From the moment we wake up each day each of us is deluged with a barrage of sensual stimuli. We often find ourselves preoccupied with the world around us. We spend the greater part of our waking time, and all too often our sleeping time as well, dealing with it, buying it, selling it, wearing it, listening to it, eating it, watching it, and other-wise trying to secure it for ourselves, or trying to secure our place in it.

T'ai Chi teaches us that there is another world, equally vast, and equally important...the world within.

In Taoism it is said that whatever is outside is also inside. If we spend our lives speeding down the highway, how much will we miss at life's roadside? The slow motion approach of T'ai Chi doesn't just allow, but rather compels, an enhanced state of self-awareness. T'ai Chi Ch'uan students learn to cultivate two important concomitant states, those of attention and intention, combining them into an inseparable "One". This facilitates personal clarity and allows us to proceed through life in a more conscious, deliberate, and enriching manner. As such, these are important "ingredients" in evolving towards better health and towards a sense of feeling more fully integrated as human beings.

As appealing as all this may sound, the real challenge is to do it right, because practicing incorrectly will fail to produce the full range of desired results. In order to learn T'ai Chi well, and derive all the aforementioned benefits, one must have a suitable guide and be prepared to commit to regular practice. T'ai Chi Ch'uan is indeed delightful to watch. Even just observing someone practice the T'ai Chi form can induce a feeling of calm and wonder. But that which is truly important in T'ai Chi is typically beyond the casual observer's perceptive abilities. It is the internal experience of T'ai Chi which is so valuable and which can prove so elusive.

> Navigating the process of learning T'ai Chi's internal subtleties is one that requires a qualified teacher. In this regard there is no shortcut.

T'ai Chi Ch'uan can certainly be many things to many people, but one thing it will do for anybody who practices it is slow them down, even if just for the duration of practice. At the very least, it serves as a model for reprieve from the out of control pace of modern life. As one flows through the slow and gentle movements of the Tai Chi sequence, the whole psycho-physiological system (the *body/mind*) relaxes (parasympathetic response), including the cardiovascular, nervous and endocrine systems. Notably, this produces a rejuvenating effect rather then a dulling of the mind or body as one might expect with such a deep level of relaxation. Surely in relaxing the body/mind and calming the spirit, T'ai Chi is, at the most basic level, an oasis for modern humankind from many of the stresses and distractions of life in today's world.

THINGS TO REMEMBER,

- Ch'i, or Life Force Energy, animates us as living beings.
- T'ai Chi body conditioning increases your range of motion while improving muscle tone and resilience.
- The Inner Structure of T'ai Chi facilitates a mechanical advantage in movement or stillness.
- Being In the Moment compels enhanced self-awareness and integration.

Notes

1. The term used throughout this book in reference to one's fuller self is "body/mind."

CHAPTER 2

Ch'i, Where Life Begins

Buried deep within, I am the Life Force
Stirring, pulsing, growing, forcing its way
Down to legs rooted in the earth,
Rising fountain-like to spine and arms,
Forming images of
Dragon writhing,
Waves rolling,
Buddha rocking.
Ch'i, be life, harmony, grace;
Be oneness, love and Spirit.
        —Sister Alice Brennan

Ch'i is the Primordial Force. It is the universal energy. It is movement, light, sound, and heat. It is Life, it is the flow of life, and it reaches beyond life. It is all encompassing. Ch'i and its manifestations are the 10,000 things spoken of by Lao Tzu.

WHY THE WEST IS PLAYING CATCH-UP—DOUBLE BLIND, OR JUST BLIND

Having said this, and with all due respect to Taoist esoterica, let us take a more practical approach, one that allows us to understand and appreciate the role of Ch'i in our daily lives. To understand Ch'i, one needs first to have an open mind and be *willing* to understand Ch'i. The idea or concept of Ch'i has been challenging on many levels to the analytical western mind so typically schooled in the need for determinable and quantifiable cause and effect. "Seeing is believing," "healthy skepticism," and especially the highly touted "double blind" research model are all representative of ideals rooted in western science and medicine's most basic premise. The most basic premise of western science and medicine is one that is both mechanistic and reductionist, a.k.a. ratio-

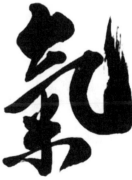

Figure 2-1. "Chi"[1]

nalism. Inherent in this approach is the belief or assumption that all things (the 10,000 things mind you) can be understood, controlled, reproduced, and (presumably) bought and sold if only they could be dismantled or dissected down to

9

their component parts, and then reassembled intact. The secret of life itself remains always just a few research dollars away.

This rationalist premise may apply on a small scale, and it does work marvelously well in many ways. It has, in fact, produced its own 10,000 things. Many of them to the genuine betterment of mankind, from Velcro to household appliances to space shuttles, or in the case of medicine, from antibiotics to heart trans-

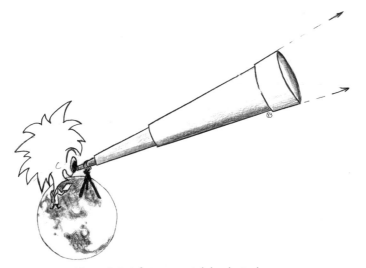

Figure 2-2. Infinite potential, but limited scope.

plants to trauma care. The problem with this western premise, despite its apparent success, is that it is just plain wrong to the extent that it sees no limits to itself. The results of this way of thinking offer infinite potential yet remain sorely limited in their scope (see Figure 2-2).

It is easy to get caught up in the idea that we live in the best of times. Life is indeed good, perhaps never better. The typical middle class American today enjoys a higher standard of living than did most world leaders prior to the Industrial Revolution. We have been to the moon and we have harnessed the atom. Yet a whole slew of problems have been either introduced or exacerbated. A sampling of these problems would include iatrogenic illness, lifestyle associated illnesses, air and water pollution, various other environmental toxins, etc. These are problems for which modern western science and medicine are directly responsible.

In addition, other issues of major import have eluded resolution, or simply not been addressed by modern science: global conflict/war, violations of human rights, racism, hunger and all the problems adjunct globally to an exploding world population, etc. More esoterically, can modern science say with any certainty what happens after death, or before life? Do we understand human nature, or the nature of being human? These are all examples of issues that western science and medicine can only ever begin to dwell on, issues that elude a rational model based solely on mechanics and reductionism.

This mechanistic/reductionist[1] view has been traditionally shortsighted to the point of arrogance. It perceives its own reality as an exclusive realm and brooks no other models of reality as viable.

> Tolerance is that quality that allows us to accept, if not respect or agree with, any rights and beliefs of others which do not encroach on our own rights or beliefs.

It is the (in)tolerance of the mechanistic/reductionist model and its historical exclusivity, which make it most wrong. In all fairness though, a new breed of western scientist seems to be emerging from this shadow. Certainly, it is possible to not endorse something and to be in total disagreement, but yet not be intolerant of it. Suffice it to say that belief systems, whether personal or institutionalized, are like stress (See Chapter on Stress) in that they get stored away in those places where they are held dear and are least likely to be challenged on their merits.

Tai Chi, on the other hand, as one manifestation of Eastern thought, is influenced by the Tao and by an understanding (resulting from observations of nature), that all things are somehow connected. Thus, there are no coincidences. All things under Heaven have a meaning and a purpose and should be respected for such. Ironically, this empiricism embodies the idea of cause and effect at its purest. The T'ai Chi model of thought, though it may have its own way of looking at things, is not based on exclusivity. Lacking its own version of the double blind model, eastern thought tends to be more empirical, and yet remarkably effective, not to mention generous, in its contributions to science and medicine. Chinese physicians were the first to discover the circulation of blood and the circadian rhythms of the body, and were responsible for the development of acupuncture—all this centuries before Christ walked the earth. Prior to the western Dark Ages, the Chinese were already prescribing for diabetes, using thyroid hormone to treat goiter, and inoculating for smallpox.[2] Indeed, the modern western model, though effective in many ways, has had no monopoly on science and medicine.

THE ROLE OF CH'I IN OUR LIVES

It is important to understand that Ch'i, though a constant universal presence, is not static. It has myriad manifestations, even insofar as its role in our being human. Of particular concern for our species are the Ch'i essences which influence and govern all aspects of our lives. The first of these is pre-birth Ch'i, (see Figure 2-3a) also known as *Yuan Ch'i* or Original Ch'i, which is bequeathed to us in finite quantities. The second is post-birth Ch'i, which we can continually manufacture within certain limits, according to our needs as we move through life (see Figures 2-3b, c).

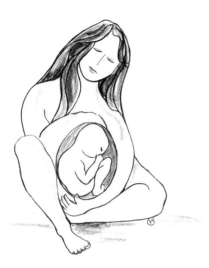

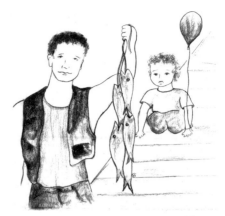

Figure 2-3b. ...becomes augmented by post-birth Chi through healthy living...

Figure 2-3a. Original Chi starts in the womb...

In the case of pre-birth Ch'i we are born with a fixed amount. That amount is determined by factors such as genetics and heredity, prenatal circumstances, and, of course, the ubiquitous Tao. All bodily functions, and in fact, our very existence, remain dependent on Original Ch'i because once it has been exhausted we have reached the end of the line, so to speak. Drug abuse, poor diet, wild living, sexual excess, or in fact, any kind of excess, all serve to deplete our store of Original Ch'i. As regards Original Ch'i, our best policy is one of *preservation of capital,*

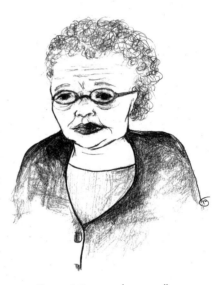

Figure 2-3c. ...and eventually declines as we age.

to borrow a term from the financial world. The best way to avoid drawing unnecessarily on our reserve of Original Ch'i is to avoid excesses of living and to maintain a balanced reserve of post-birth Ch'i.

Post-birth Ch'i is available to us via healthy living, which includes healthy food and drink, sufficient sleep, balanced exercise, and generally living in harmony with the Tao. We actually manufacture this Ch'i according to our needs. Notably, disciplines such as T'ai Chi Ch'uan, Ch'i Kung, and energy oriented meditation practices can serve to augment our post-birth Ch'i. One of the functions of post-birth Ch'i is that of defense. This Ch'i is known as protective Ch'i or *Wei Ch'i.*

This *Wei Ch'i* is of particular concern to T'ai Chi'ers and martial artists in general because it can be cultivated through T'ai Chi practice and Ch'i Kung exercises to the point where it can actually "insulate" the body, rendering it more resilient and less vulnerable to injury. *Wei Ch'i*, when strong, can extend beyond the shell of the physical body, (as has been evidenced by Kirlian photography.) In fact *Wei Ch'i* is very much like the energy deflector shield on the Starship Enterprise (see Figure 2-4). It plays a leading role in the efficacy of the body's immune response, functioning as a first line of defense against invasion by *evil and pernicious influences* (as pathological influences are referred to in TCM). Anybody who has cultivated a strong *Wei Ch'i* function will be less susceptible to illness or injury and will recover more quickly should illness or injury occur. A strong *Wei Ch'i* function also serves to maintain, or restore, a youthful vitality.

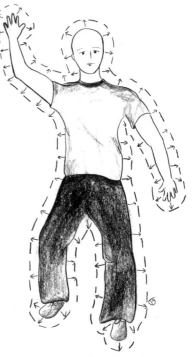

Figure 2-4. Wei Chi is like a force field which can be developed to insulate the body from illness and injury.

T'AI CHI AND SEX

One other manifestation of Ch'i that begs mention is that of Jing, or sexual essence. (How could any book in this day and age be written without the obligatory mention of SEX?) This is a topic of some controversy even in the internal arts community where many feel the discussion or dissemination of opinions and teachings pertaining to sex is in poor taste, or at best, of questionable value. Many teachers simply fail to see the connection. As it relates to Ch'i and T'ai Chi, the issue of sex is no less or more important than any other topic covered in this book; it is simply one important component of a larger whole. As such, it should not be ignored. I would emphasize however, the absence of any prurient quality in this context.

Sexual energy is the most powerful and influential energy available to us as living beings in that it alone allows us to reproduce ourselves as a species. Traditional Chinese Medicine (TCM) views a moderate amount of sexual activity as not unhealthy. However, by many standards, sexual excess is rampant today, though in all likelihood it probably always has been in one form or another throughout the ages. If history is any indication, the mere repression of sexual energy appears not to dampen its need for expression. My view is that rather than opting for either extreme, that of repressing sexual energy versus that of leaving it wild and unchecked, its expression can be moderated and/or re-channeled. If done properly, this approach can serve as a basis for personal growth on many levels.

The significance of *Jing* as it relates to T'ai Chi, lies in the fact that (for men) the kidneys are understood to store the sexual essence. The kidneys are further understood to govern the bones, their health and strength, and their exact articulation, which are all critical to T'ai Chi development. Sexual excess will not only deplete the kidneys and thus weaken the bones, it will undermine the integrity of the aforementioned *Wei Ch'i* function as well. Male T'ai Chi players, who also happen to be sexual spendthrifts, will find sooner or later that they are taking two steps back for every step forward. Increasingly men are seeking out T'ai Chi as a means of addressing the issue of lower back pain, an issue that can certainly be caused or exacerbated by sexual excess. Lest women feel excluded from this topic, let me hasten to add that unlike men, women are not at risk of depleting sexual essence through sexual activity. (Women are more at risk for depleting sexual energy via menstruation and childbirth.)

Two excellent books available on the subject that I recommend for those wishing to learn more about managing sexual energy are *Healing Love Through the Tao* (for women) and *Taoist Secrets of Love* (for men), both available at your bookstore or through the Healing Tao Press.[3]

CH'I: SUBJECTIVE VERSUS OBJECTIVE

The intangible nature of C'hi, more than any other factor, probably best explains the late wakeup call for the West when it came to recognizing the existence of Ch'i energy. As noted earlier, Ch'i defies even exact definition let alone quantification. Consequently, any experience of Ch'i tends to be more subjective than objective. This puts the very existence of C'hi in diametric opposition to the western model of mechanics and reduction, premised as it is on identification and categorization. That which cannot be identified and quantified cannot fruitfully be reduced to its component parts. No microscope or telescope alone will get us any closer to understanding—or exploiting—the essence of Ch'i.

USING INTENTION TO CULTIVATE CH'I

Each and every one of us already has Ch'i energy regardless of whether or not we feel it. It is this "Life Force Energy" that animates each of us as living beings. One curious aspect of working with Ch'i, which simply adds to the confusion for western science and medicine, is the manner in which it responds to subjective rather than objective stimuli. In the case of C'hi, intention is a critical variable. This is why double blind research models are so limited in their application to more fully understand, or even just validate, the existence of Ch'i. All other factors being equal, those individuals who have the clearest intention are usually the ones best able to consciously experience their energy. A truly skeptical person (one lacking a genuine intention) cannot be made to experience any manifestation of his or her own energy in the absence of third party intervention. Certainly a Ch'i Kung healer, or an acupuncturist, can apply healing energies to a skeptical subject. These are energies that the unwilling subject may or may not actually feel. But there is still the subjective intention of the source behind the energy. Intention and some element of belief or acceptance inherent in that intention are thus necessary ingredients in the cultivation of Ch'i.

USING ATTENTION TO CULTIVATE CH'I

Many westerners are additionally challenged in cultivating Ch'i despite their intention to do so. In this case, the missing variable may be one of attention. I do not believe it is an overstatement to say that there is a cultural disincentive for us to pay attention to what goes on inside ourselves given the western propensity for indulging in and being deluged by sensual stimuli (see Figure 2-5). The Five Thieves (the five senses), as they are known in eastern cultures, have been the downfall of many an otherwise well-intentioned practitioner. Unless you can at least manage, if not curb, sensual over-stimu-

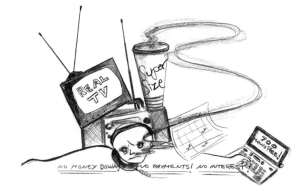

Figure 2-5. Sensory overload can be burdensome to the point that it distracts us from being mindfully attentive to our own inner process.

lation you will never be able to achieve the state of mindfulness necessary to manage your energy on a deeper level. The best approach then, to cultivating your own Ch'i, is one in which you are able to combine a clear intention and belief with a focused attention. If you can do that then you should achieve good results regardless of which of the innumerable Ch'i cultivation techniques you adopt for your own practice.

WHY GO TO ALL THAT EFFORT TO CULTIVATE CH'I?

In answering this question it may be helpful to first understand just what factors prompted the development of the genre of Ch'i cultivation practices in the first place. In their regard for what happens after death, the Taoist sages were no different from the seekers of many other religions or spiritual traditions. The Taoists believed they could achieve immortality and were ambitious in their pursuit toward that end. The problem though, was that the spiritual cultivation necessary to become Immortal (allegedly) took a great deal of time, more so than was often available in a typical life span. The obvious solution to this dilemma was to live longer and thus have more time and opportunity to complete the requisite preparation. T'ai Chi and many of the various Ch'i Kung practices proved ideal adjuncts to this greater task in that they served both to enhance the quality of life in the here and now and to promote one's health and longevity towards the pursuit of immortality.

Regardless of its form or manifestation, all Ch'i has an inherent polarity, roughly analogous to that of electricity. This is denoted by the terms yin and yang (versus negative and positive) that must be kept in balance. As each of us moves through life growing older we begin to deplete our pre-birth Ch'i and our energy begins to polarize. This polarization process can be exacerbated by less than healthy lifestyles and by the various kinds of trauma: illness, injury, disease, loss, anxiety, etc. which we all inevitably experience from time to time to the detriment of our health and well-being. Left unchecked, this process will contribute to disharmony/dis-ease and can further accelerate our own aging process both qualitatively and quantitatively in a terminal spiral. Few, if any, of us will likely achieve the fabled immortality sought by the Taoists. However, by committing ourselves to a regular and ongoing practice of T'ai Chi we can begin to curb the effects of those factors in our lives that would undermine our health or upset the balance of our own personal energy. Thus we can use our T'ai Chi in a practical way to correct existing imbalances as well as to diminish or prevent the occurrence or effects of future imbalances.

YOU AND YOUR CH'I

It is commonly the case that students new to T'ai Chi or other internal disciplines are prompted in their studies by a desire to learn more about their own energy. Given the significance of the aforementioned "subjective intent" in pursuing energy work such as T'ai Chi, there is no one standard measure by which anyone can determine their own progress, or lack thereof, when it comes to energy cultivation. In fact, students who are at a practice level where their experience of Ch'i energy tends to be more transient and less predictably replicable may even find themselves wondering if the whole business of energy is not just in their imagination. Other than a telltale visible mottling of the palms (which can certainly occur due to other causes) there are very few external or objective indicators that one's Ch'i is manifesting at all.

Based on my own experience in working with students of energy oriented practices I can share the following information in order to shed some light on commonly asked questions about Ch'i. Probably the most common question I am asked is, "What does Ch'i feel like?" The actual experience of Ch'i can vary widely from person to person, and for any given person at different times. Most people *feel* their energy, perhaps as a (somewhat indescribable) wave, or they may feel it as a tingling sensation, or thermally (as heat and/or coolness), or as a feeling of expansion/contraction (either, or even both simultaneously). Some people tend to *see* their energy as a light or color, while others may *hear* their energy as a frequency, a tone or a buzz.

The area of the body where one senses one's energy can also vary. The most common places for Ch'i to be felt are the head, genitals, dantien, feet, or spine. The most common place for T'ai Chi'ers to sense Ch'i energy are the hands and fingers. This is due to the concentration of attention/intention on the exact positioning and function of the hands during form practice.

It is also true that the quality or quantity of your energy can be more or less available according to stressors or distractions present in your life. Generally though, less experienced practitioners tend to experience more unpredictable variations in energy levels. Ongoing and correct practice will tend to moderate this tendency toward energy extremes, as the effects of energy disciplines such as T'ai Chi or Ch'i Kung, are usually cumulative over time. Bearing this in mind, your own practice of whatever discipline you choose, should be regular and frequent in order to obtain good results.

CULTIVATING YOUR CH'I, THINGS TO CONSIDER

There are enough different teachers teaching enough different techniques for cultivating Ch'i that I will not add to that list in this chapter. (Directions for a simple Standing Ch'i Kung practice are provided in Chapter 7.)

I personally have studied more Ch'i Kung practices over the last thirty-five years than I care to remember, let alone am able to remember. There is certainly a wealth of books and audiovisual resources available to anyone who wants to learn more about the cultivation of Ch'i. Unless you are gifted and naturally oriented toward mindful work, I recommend you seek out a qualified teacher or guide.

As I see it, there are three important variables for you to take into consideration.

The first variable has to do with which technique or method you choose to practice. Though some techniques may be more ideally suited for you based on your agenda or your state of health and fitness, any credible technique can produce good results.

The second variable is the quality of instruction. This can be quite important as a good instructor will be able to present his or her teachings in a way that renders the work relevant to you, factoring in your particular learning style. He or she will also be able to intervene on your behalf with corrections, cautionary advice, and encouragement. Bearing this in mind, you should seek out someone with whom you can establish a comfortable level of trust and rapport. I recommend that you feel free to experiment with different teachers or techniques if you do not get some sense of progress after a reasonable effort has been made. Of course, what constitutes a "reasonable effort" can depend on a number of variables. You might find it helpful to discuss the issues of expectations and goals with your teacher at the onset of your training, and again at various intervals throughout.

This will give you a guideline for recognizing any progress or personal shifts as a result of your practice.

The third, final, and most important variable is what you bring to the table. Of course this includes any pre-existing health issues, but it is more a matter of you having what it takes to do the work. No matter who the teacher is, or what the technique, you must assume a clear responsibility as regards attention/intention, commitment to doing your practice, and above all, making a commitment to the process. At the same time, you must be aware that this process may include setbacks or even failure(s) en route. In the absence of such a commitment, you will fall short of achieving the desired results. In order to get good results you must do your work, keeping in mind that results are cumulative over time and often subtle beyond your expectations.

THINGS TO REMEMBER
- The T'ai Chi model of thought is not based on exclusivity.
- Our existence depends on Original Ch'i. Once it's gone, we're gone.
- We can augment our Original Ch'i with Post-Birth Ch'i through healthy living.
- A strong *Wei Ch'i* function serves to maintain or restore youthful vitality.
- Chi responds to subjective stimuli. Thus "Intention" is a critical variable.
- The effects of energy cultivation practices such as T'ai Chi or Ch'i Kung are cumulative over time. Regular correct practice produces the best results.

Notes
1. The character for "ch'i" is courtesy of Master Wei Lun Huang.

2. Rationalism is commonly ascribed to the 17th century philosopher/scientist René Descartes, but in actuality dates back to the Greek Parmenides circa 500 B.C.

3. Robert Temple. *The Genius of China.* 1989

4. Both books by Mantak Chia.

CHAPTER 3

Understanding Stress as It Relates to T'ai Chi

Complete freedom from stress is death.
—Hans Selye. M.D.

(Note: Notwithstanding the venerable Dr. Selye's definition of stress cited above, I have opted to use this term in its vernacular sense, that of stress connotatively understood to mean dis-stress.)

T'ai Chi is beautiful to watch, soft and fluid in its appearance. It can present an almost hypnotic quality in its effect on the casual observer. Visitors sitting in on classes at my school often remark afterwards that just watching a T'ai Chi class has left them feeling more relaxed and less stressed. With increasing frequency, T'ai Chi is being sought out and marketed based on its reputation as a stress reducer. T'ai Chi can be marvelously effective in this regard because of its emphasis on integration (versus dis-integration) of body and mind.

For many people, T'ai Chi presents its own unique set of challenges, often stemming from the very same factors (feelings of stress, etc.) that may have led them to T'ai Chi in the first place. Beginners at T'ai Chi reasonably start off with a vision, or perhaps a goal, of acquiring some level of skill at T'ai Chi in order to be better off eventually than they were before undertaking their new studies. In order to derive the full range of benefits that T'ai Chi has to offer, students need, eventually, to get beyond the mere superficialities of memorizing the T'ai Chi form routine. They must "get it right" regarding such issues as posture and carriage, weight distribution and rooting, and fluidity and balance. Every T'ai Chi student aspires to eventual proficiency in these areas. But it is the "getting there" that counts, and it is important to understand that getting it right is actually more of a process itself than it is a goal. The first step in that process is to begin by addressing any long held psycho/somatic issues such as stress, tension, and anxiety lest one's best efforts be thwarted by the body/mind itself.

HOW STRESS AFFECTS THE BODY/MIND

To better understand why this is important, you need to understand how stress affects the body/mind. Currently, there is a great deal of information available dealing with the relationships between stress and genetic predisposition, neurochemistry, lifestyle influences and psychopharmacology, etc. These cutting edge fields are changing rapidly with new discoveries and advances. However fascinating it may be to keep abreast of new developments in science and medicine, for the purpose of this topic a rudimentary understanding of how the body/mind responds to stressors will suffice.

The body/mind's autonomic nervous system, which controls among other things its involuntary functions, is comprised of two branches, the sympathetic branch and the parasympathetic branch (see Figure 3-1). Briefly, the sympathetic branch controls the "fight or flight response" while the parasympathetic branch oversees the body/mind's "relaxation response." (An easy way to remember how to distinguish between the two is to imagine falling out of an airplane. If you are wearing a *para*chute you can relax, otherwise you will deserve some *sym*pathy.) When confronted with any danger the sympathetic response is acute and powerful. Capillaries dilate, digestion slows and breathing becomes more rapid. This response is one of the body/mind's primary natural survival mechanisms and is well designed for response to any threat, real or imagined.

It has long been understood that activation of the sympathetic branch of the nervous system can be caused by non life-threatening stress and tension. A problem for many people though, is that just living their lives is stressful. This puts the sympathetic nervous system's response into overdrive, triggering a chronic excitation of the body/mind's fight or flight response. It literally forgets how to turn itself off. This in turn exacerbates disunity and disconnection from the earth and creates a self-perpetuating downward spiral. This downward spiral prevents the body/mind from being able to discriminate in its responses to the different sources of stress.

The upshot is that most people carry some degree of chronic stress in their body/mind. This makes complete relaxation difficult if not impossible, because no one can carry stress and be completely relaxed at the same time. Paradoxically, a person can *be* stressed and not *feel* stressed. Once stress has been committed to the body/mind for any length of time the "self" may well desensitize to the point that that person can lose any conscious awareness of underlying stress. Thus, people often operate

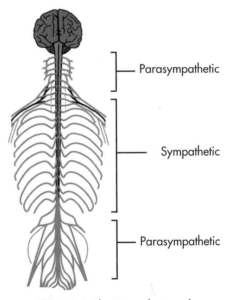

Parasympathetic

Sympathetic

Parasympathetic

Figure 3-1. The Sympathetic and Parasympathetic branches of the Autonomic Nervous System.

under the delusion that they are relaxed when in fact they are not. T'ai Chi has a way of revealing this to those who practice it.

One of the more fascinating aspects of my chosen role as a martial arts instructor is being a body watcher. Everybody's body has a story to tell. I use what I observe in bodies to teach people about themselves in a way that makes a real difference in their lives. I have frequently revealed obvious postural imbalances to students who were blissfully unaware of postural problems such as tilted alignment, raised shoulders, uneven hips, etc. They had never even considered the possibility of postural problems until I stood them in front of a mirror and said, "There, does that look straight to you?" So the very first order of business is to identify if and where problem areas exist. Only then can you begin to address these areas in any comprehensive manner.

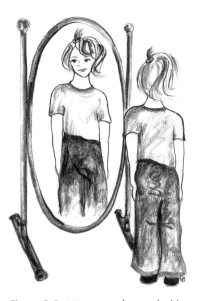

Figure 3-2. Mirrors can be invaluable, albeit brutally honest, in revealing postural imbalances.

RELEASING VERSUS RELINQUISHING STRESS

The next step is to begin to release, or more accurately relinquish, stress and tension from the body/mind. Releasing stress is pretty easy: you take a few deep breaths, or you kick back and relax, perhaps in a hot tub (see Figure 3-3), or simply remove yourself from the source of stress. This need not be a big deal. Case in point: I recall, as I sat trying to write this very chapter, rewriting it for the umpteenth time in an effort to produce my best work, when I realized I was working way too hard at it. So I put it down and walked away for a bit. Just this simple act cleared the clutter from my mind's surface and allowed me to continue afresh. These and other simple little tricks are sometimes all that's needed to afford at least a modicum of relief from the immediacies of feeling stressed.

"Relinquishing" stress however, is different from releasing stress, and can itself be a daunting task. Once stress has been stored in the body/mind it gets held there indefinitely, and then proceeds to accumulate in layers over time with repeated exposure to other stressors. There are "special places" (which may be specific to the individual or to the stressor) in the body and mind both that are like the proverbial closets into which all the junk gets tossed. The reason for this response to stress is that it is not some separate "thing" or entity distinct from us. Stress is the body/mind's self-generated response to any perceived demand for which it is not optimally prepared to cope. "Stress" is actually a survival mechanism and the manifestation of unresolved conflict in the body/mind. It is the body/mind's best effort to protect itself, to act in what it believes to be its own best interests at all times. In just a short bit I will guide you through a very simple exercise that you can use to identify, and then begin to relinquish, stress from your own body/mind.

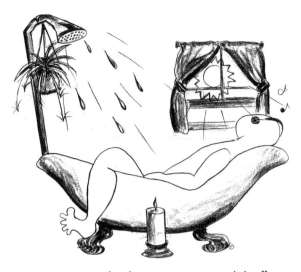

Figure 3-3. Simple relaxation requires very little effort.

STRESS AS AN INVESTMENT

The problem with our response to stress is that while the body/mind is marvelously capable of creating stress, ostensibly to protect itself, this response is physiologically primitive, lacking any intelligent capacity for discrimination. We are as likely to feel stressed over getting stuck in traffic as we are being held up at gun point. Once the body/mind has been taxed beyond its ability to manage stressors effectively, it will have become conditioned to simply store new stress. It will continue to accumulate layer upon layer until and unless provided with some incentive to do otherwise. Incentives to *do otherwise* can be generated by third party intervention or self-generated from within, the latter being rare indeed. This is because once the body/mind has acted in its own interest by creating stress, it is loathe to let it go, even if the original stressors are no longer present.

When it comes to stress, "Easy come, easy go," does not apply, and most people end up living out their lives unaware of the depth of the stress they carry (see Figure 3-4). Stress held in the body/mind becomes in effect an investment. As it is a truism in the world of finance that nobody likes to consciously acknowledge, even to themselves, that they have made a bad investment, so it is with the body/mind. Recall the example I described about standing a student in front of a mirror (a reliable source of brutally honest feedback) where she could see clearly for herself that one shoulder was riding higher than the other. In such a circumstance I can always expect that after repositioning the shoulder and eliciting both recognition and approval from my subject, the same shoulder will invariably return to its known, albeit unbalanced, position within the next minute or so, as soon as the attention being focused on the shoulder is drawn elsewhere. Likewise, the body/mind holds its stress, reluctant to relinquish it lest it be left exposed and vulnerable to some new and unknown danger. The known danger is always safer and more predictable than the unknown. Consequently, you will not want to exacerbate stress that you may already have stored in your body by embarking on any course of action that the body/mind might perceive as being in conflict with the stress it is already invested in.

DIVESTING YOURSELF OF STRESS AND TENSION HELD IN THE BODY

Let us try the following experiment to see how stress and tension can first be identified and then released a bit. You will need to find a willing partner, preferably someone with obvious stress. Have your partner stand straight, feet slightly apart, hands and arms relaxed down. Begin by asking your partner to

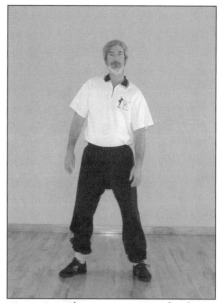

Figure 3-4. Chronic stress accumulated over time can wreak insidious havoc with your body. The photo above depicts a badly misaligned body. Note the oblique foot alignment and the shoulders out of level, even as the head compensates in its best effort to remain properly upright.

extend one arm to the front at about shoulder height, employing the least possible amount of effort to do so (see Figure 3-5). Now ask your partner, and any observers present, to note how relaxed he appears to be, and how relaxed his arm actually feels. After you have done this, your partner can lower his arm back down by his side.

In the next step, as your partner tries to refrain from any involvement whatso-ever, you will raise his arm for him, lifting it up to the same shoulder height posi-tion as before. His challenge will be to simply let go completely, surrendering ownership of that arm to you. If he manages to stay relaxed, his arm should feel loose and quite heavy, like a dead weight. Unless you have a subject who is natu-rally relaxed or already skilled at T'ai Chi, he will probably try unconsciously to help out as you raise his arm. Each time you feel his arm tighten or lighten, drop it down a bit as a reminder to him to let go and relax. A truly relaxed arm will drop like a bag of cement. Anything short of this means your partner has failed to relinquish his arm completely. In this case, gently coax him to just let go (see Figure 3-6). Relaxing, in the context of this exercise, can take some real effort and concentration. Relinquishment of stress and tension can seem real work at first.

Once you have managed to get your partner's relaxed arm back up to shoulder height, tell him you are about to slowly remove your supporting hands in order to

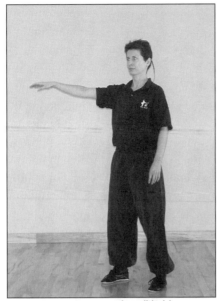

Figure 3-5. Most people will hold tension even in an arm they believe to be relaxed.

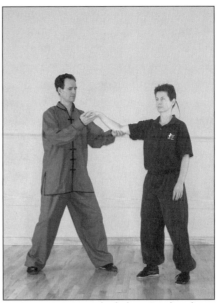

Figure 3-6. Here the helper coaches the subject to relax her arm by providing support at her wrist and elbow.

see if he is able to continue to hold his arm aloft and still remain soft. Then slowly proceed to do so. If he has relaxed and truly let go, the difference to him in the feeling of his arm and the difference in its appearance to any observers should be obvious to all present when compared with his earlier attempt to relax (see Figure 3-7).

This exercise will clearly illustrate that for your partner, as for most people, the body/mind unwittingly engages to a much greater extent than is necessary to accomplish even the simplest of tasks. Bear in mind that this is just an exercise, a first step in revealing the presence and impact of underlying stress and tension.

If you have a regular practice partner, or if you are a teacher working with students, you can make this exercise an occasional part of your practice. Remember, the greater part of stress and

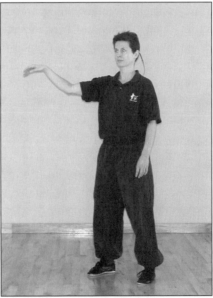

Figure 3-7. Having released unnecessary tension through the guidance of her coach, the subject can now relax her arm, expending a bare minimum amount of effort to hold it aloft once support has been removed.

tension held in the body is there because the body/mind has become conditioned to holding it so. But conditioning works both ways. Over time you will notice that by practicing with just this simple exercise you can (re)condition the body/mind to relinquish stress and tension to the point that you become able to relax on demand. Of course, it is best to start with small areas that can serve as models for working with other parts of the body, in time working up to the body/mind as a fuller entity.

UNDERSTANDING WHAT YOU ARE UP AGAINST

In order for the body to relinquish long held stresses, it must first be presented with repeated and convincing incentives to change its patterns. Acting on your best intention in responding to perceived stress you may try, for example, a stretching session to relieve chronically tightened muscles, or perhaps going for a run to jog anxiety away from a stressed out body/mind. But the body/mind may well perceive your efforts as one more assault to be defended against by further bolstering its defenses, allowing you, at best, to release superficial layers of stress, yet leaving the deeper underlying stresses intact.

> This is important to understand because any effort made at relinquishing the body/mind's chronic stress is likely to put one at cross purposes with one's deeper or unconscious self. In conflicts between the conscious self and the unconscious self, the unconscious self will usually manage to prevail.

This is so because in the primitive hierarchy between conscious and unconscious mind the unconscious always enjoys the last word. The trick is to "outsmart" the unconscious self by avoiding any appearance of conflict. If you can learn to do this then you will have at your disposal an effective means of relinquishing stress and tension.

KNOW WHEN TO GET HELP

This means that one of the first orders of business in T'ai Chi is to begin to address those factors that prevent or interfere with your being fully relaxed, but in a way that does not excite further stress. Let me hasten to add here that relaxation in T'ai Chi is conscious and deliberate and is not to be confused with being limp or sedentary. Being relaxed and being limp are two entirely different qualities. (So, kicking back on the sofa and napping do not qualify as T'ai Chi relaxation techniques!)

Exactly how your own various stresses are best addressed is contingent on your perception of them. People who perceive their stress to be harbored primarily in the psyche may seek out therapy of one sort or another. (Note: In some cases medication may be called for. Though I am not an enthusiastic advocate for psycho-pharmaceutical medication, I do recognize its propriety as an interim solution when called for.) Others, who experience their stress more somatically, might try mindful exercise or therapeutic bodywork. I AM a big proponent of other adjunctive therapies to catalyze change, therapies such as deep tissue massage, chiropractic, psychotherapy, acupuncture, and homeopathy among others. Adjuncts such as these can prove invaluable in helping the body/mind to relinquish long held issues. Remember, you want to avoid any perception of working at cross-purposes with your own body/mind. Intervention by a skilled and objective third party can streamline this process.

Having said this, there are very effective ways that you can begin to use T'ai Chi to address these issues as well. I credit my teacher of recent years, Master Wei Lun Huang, with revolutionizing my own T'ai Chi experience. After a lifetime of hard driven external martial arts, and despite my extensive T'ai Chi training up until I began to work with Master Huang, the body part of my body/mind was entering into a dis-integration phase. I found myself relying with increasing frequency on visits to my chiropractor or massage therapist to address annoying lapses in my body's integrity. I had become the perfect example of someone who was using ostensibly healthy activities (i.e. external style martial arts, racquet sports, running, and other high impact sports) to unwittingly aggravate deeply held stresses accumulated over many years.

USING T'AI CHI TO RELINQUISH STRESS

Master Huang's approach, which I have adopted into my own practice, was (is) brilliant in its simplicity. His approach emphasizes the opening and conditioning of the body on a very deep level, that of the bones, tendons, joints, and connective tissues, versus the muscles, per se. The secret is to start small with any given exercise, beginning slowly and gently so the body/mind's initial reaction is not one of alarm. As you begin any particular exercise maintain a conscious synchronicity with the breath, only gradually increasing the scope or range of motion, as well as any other demands on the body/mind inherent in that particular exercise. Using this approach the body/mind is lulled into a more relaxed and secure place, where disarmament of preexisting defense mechanisms is met with little or no resistance. In this manner, the natural tendency of the body to retrench and resist change is rendered less counterproductive, if not eliminated altogether, over time.

This is one effective means by which stress can be gradually relinquished in order to allow one actually to feel progress being made towards improved T'ai Chi and overall health. In my own case, as well as that of many of my students, I have found this approach (to improve flexibility by relaxing, versus stretching, muscles) to work remarkably well. Even more impressive is the improvement in soft tissue resilience, which is the body's ability to withstand and recover quickly from the extraordinary demands of intensive practice sessions. In this sense my body feels as young at age forty-seven as it did when I was thirty-five.

This method is also a great way to get the body/mind warmed up, in order to derive optimal benefit, prior to a session of form practice. Bear in mind, however, the word "warm-up" is itself a misnomer. In my T'ai Chi classes warm-ups are not something done simply to prepare for something else, such as form practice or pushing hands. Rather, this preparation phase is an integral part of the T'ai Chi learning experience. The principles described in the previous paragraph can be applied to render just about any preparation work deeper and more effective in relinquishing stress.

This would be an ideal place for me to insert directions for some exercise that readers could try at home in order to illustrate my point. However, experience has taught me that a live, or at least audiovisual, context is best for learning the particular method just described. Following the lead of a skilled guide is really the only way you can practice exercises in a way that allows you to divest yourself of old patterns. Otherwise you will probably just be reinforcing preexisting problems without even realizing it. Ideally, you should seek out a competent T'ai Chi instructor and entrust yourself to his or her guidance. Try to find someone who is skilled enough to be able to recognize and affect changes in those areas of your own body where stresses and tensions reveal themselves as postural imbalances or inadequate rooting skills. For advice on how to find a qualified instructor see the Consumer's Guide chapter later in this book. However, you can practice on your own in order to become more conscientious with regard to breathing and mindfulness patterns.

CONSCIOUS ABDOMINAL BREATHING

As I mentioned earlier, one of the effects of being even in a low grade sympathetic excitation state is that breathing becomes chronically shallower. The fact that stress is endemic in our society today is one reason why so many people are chronic chest breathers. Even many individuals who get regular aerobic exercise tend to breathe in this shallow manner, utilizing only the upper portions of the lungs. Breathing shallowly reduces stamina and undermines optimal functioning of the body's immune system. It also serves to reinforce the very problems that cause it in the first place. Stress begets stress. So it is no surprise that people pay so little conscious attention to breathing. Breathing is an involuntary function. We breathe automatically, just to stay alive, and with such repetitive frequency, day in and day out, breathing hardly commands our attention.

However, the simple act of breathing consciously into your lower abdomen can have a profound effect on all of the body/mind's myriad functions. Conscious abdominal breathing induces the body/mind's relaxation response. This approach to breathing can be implemented in any number of contexts. Here is one very simple exercise you can try in order to become more aware of stress held in the body/mind and to encourage regular and proper breathing habits.

GUIDING THE BREATH

While lying flat on your back, fold your hands comfortably over your lower abdomen just below the navel. Use your mind to notice the pattern of your respiration and stay with it over two or three breaths. Gradually relax the thoracic diaphragm (the horizontal band of muscle under the lungs) and use your mind to guide your breath more deeply into the abdomen. In guiding your breath, you can visualize its passage through the nostrils, via the trachea into the lungs, under the diaphragm, and down into the lower abdomen where, as it fills the belly, you will feel the abdomen expand upwards like a cake rising (see Figure 3-8). Your hands, resting on your rising belly, will serve both as a confirmation of this process and as a means of anchoring your attention to the *Dantien* (belly) as a destination point for the breath. Hold your breath briefly, then, as you release out, you can feel the lower abdomen settle back down. In exhaling, use your mind's eye to follow the breath as you use your intention to guide it back up along the inside of the spine to the top of your head, finally venting the breath out through your nostrils (see Figure 3-9). Repeat this 6—10 times, or more as needed. Simple abdominal breathing like this can be very restful, so unless you are trying to fall asleep, be sure to remain deliberate and attentive to this process even as you relax. Guiding the breath will require some initiative on your part at first, especially if you have not practiced breathing skills in the past. Be sure you have a solid grasp of this skill to the point of its being automatic before you proceed on to try the next variation.

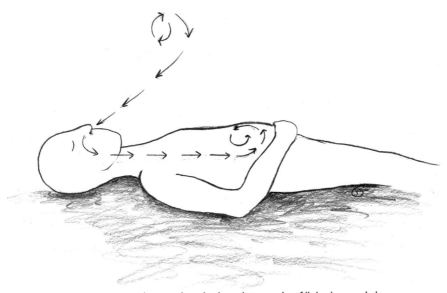

Figure 3-8. Visualize guiding the breath inward to fill the lower abdomen as shown by the arrows above.

ALLOWING THE BREATH

Once you have accustomed yourself to guiding the breath you can experiment alternately with the level of initiative you assume in "guiding" versus simply "allowing" the breath to move. In terms of its pathway through your body, the experience of merely allowing your breath to fill the abdomen is similar to the earlier version. But in comparison to the visualization and initiative of the earlier technique, this variation is more reliant on pure attention and intention than it is on any conscious effort you make to breathe. It is a fine line between doing by doing and doing by not doing. Indeed, it can be challenging at first to relinquish all initiative and just trust that your focused attention/intention will suffice to inspire an altered physiological function. But if you followed the directions in the previous section to establish a foundation in Guiding the Breath, then Allowing the Breath is a reasonable and attainable next step representing a deeper level of practice.

STRESS IN THE MIND

Just as T'ai Chi can be useful in relinquishing stress from the body, so can its practice be applied to relinquishing accumulated stress from the mind, or, of equal importance, to moderate the role of the mind in responding to stressors. Given that stress is an internal dynamic in response to internal or external stimuli, the mind often plays a key role in assigning the degree of importance to any given stressor. Often the degree of importance assigned may be based on past experience in anticipation of, or in preparation for, future experience, with little regard for

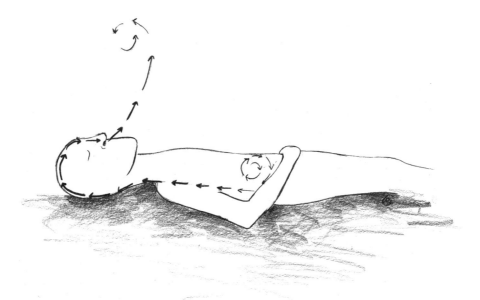

Figure 3-9. Hold briefly, then visualize releasing the breath down to and through perineum, then up the spine and out the nostrils, as shown.

the reality of the moment at hand. For example: encountering a certain person may have been stressful for you in the past. In preparing to meet the same person again you may expect and prepare for an equally stressful encounter, even before it happens. You may, in effect, *pre-create* that stress. In this way your response may be out of proportion to the reality of the presenting stressor. Certainly, many people spend a great deal of their time dwelling in, or reaching to, the past in an effort to somehow ensure a better future. When you stop to think about it, the only moment that you really have any control over is the moment you are in, right now! But you cannot influence this moment deliberately if you are not present in it. Being in the moment at hand allows you to more fully and deliberately participate in your own life. This in and of itself can help you to be and to feel more in control and less stressed.

BREATH IS LIFE

Remember, breath is life, and breathing affords us the most direct and reliable access to the Ch'i around us. Mindful breathing is also a very effective way to bring ourselves more consciously into the moment. Any time you prepare to embark on a round of T'ai Chi practice, prior to engaging your body in an active manner, take a few minutes for quiet time with some sitting or standing meditation, and then begin with a few simple conscious breaths. Each time you breathe mindfully you align yourself in a more fluid harmony with the 10,000 things, integrating with, rather than dis-integrating from, the world around you. By practicing T'ai Chi in the correct manner, you will relinquish deeply held and self-limiting stresses. You will enhance your overall quality of life, as you simultaneously create a healthier and more enduring vessel to carry you on through life.

T'AI CHI AS A RECUPERATIVE MODALITY

Aside from T'ai Chi's efficacy in addressing chronic stress held in the body/mind, it can also be useful in addressing stress of a more acute nature. This can be seen in the case of recovery from accidental injury, or from medical procedures or conditions for which controlled and non-jarring movement or exercise is indicated. T'ai Chi can be safely employed as an adjunct to recuperative therapy because its movements are by design, slow and mindful. For many patients in recovery the boundaries of previously known limits are delicate and tenuous and no longer predictably familiar. Exercise therapies that rely on faster movements may preclude the recognition of one's newer limits until after those limits are already exceeded, resulting in injury or re-injury. T'ai Chi, on the other hand, can allow one to perceive where one's limits are *as they are approached,* and to remain safely within the bounds of those limits even while challenging their constraints.

THINGS TO REMEMBER:

- Getting it right is more of a process than a goal
- A first order of business in T'ai Chi is to address stress in the body/mind.
- You cannot hold stress and be completely relaxed at the same time.
- Stress is not some separate thing. It is the body/mind's best effort to protect itself from any danger.
- You can condition the body/mind to relinquish stress and to relax on demand.
- Try to maintain a conscious synchronicity with the breath at all times. Conscious breathing induces the relaxation response to help you feel better and stay healthier.
- The only moment you really control is the moment you are in right now.
- T'ai Chi can be an excellent recuperative modality.

CHAPTER 4

The Importance of Rooting, How to Get Yours and Keep It

"You have brains in your head.
You have feet in your shoes.
You can steer yourself any direction you choose.
You're on your own, and you know what you know.
And YOU are the guy who'll decide where to go."
    —Dr. Seuss, Oh, the Places You'll Go! *(1990)*

"One small step for man, one giant step for mankind",
    —Neil Armstrong, 1969

but he had no root!
    —Author's commentary on Neil Armstrong's 1969 moon walk.

WHY ROOT?

In today's world life is rapid paced and people have for the most part, fallen out of touch with the earth. Most of us rely heavily on a diet of processed food. We rarely walk barefoot, and when we do walk it is usually over asphalt or concrete. In fact, most people would prefer to drive or catch a cab, and then only if they are unable to hop a train or catch a plane. We may jog for exercise, but usually with the idea in mind of completing a run, versus connecting mindfully with the earth. Many of the clothes we wear are made from synthetic fibers. And so it goes. Increasingly, we have moved away from direct contact with the earth. And yet, the earth is still our Mother. It still nourishes us and provides (albeit, somewhat less directly) all our basic needs. There are just more middlemen involved now than in times past. Admittedly, fast paced living does have its advantages when looked at from the perspective of productivity and the fulfillment of one's need or preference for immediate gratification. But, conversely, there is a way that a more direct and deliberate connection with the earth can soothe our souls and afford us some sense of sanity when life feels a bit out of hand. Being connected to the earth and continuing to derive the benefits of modern living are neither incompatible nor mutually exclusive dynamics. So, how then can we enjoy the best of both worlds? T'ai Chi holds an answer to this question.

WHAT IS ROOTING?

One of those qualities by which T'ai Chi practitioners are often judged is their ability to "root", or to establish and maintain a firm connection to the ground on which they stand. Rooting is quite different from merely keeping one's balance. Being "balanced" simply means being able to hold or arrange your body in such a manner as to offset the natural effects of gravity that would have us fall down. Rooting entails a much more deliberate approach to connecting with the earth than merely standing on it. Accordingly, rooting skills can be of particular benefit to older persons because of the natural decline in proprioceptive feedback that typifies the aging process. Older persons who know how to root will be much less susceptible to falling or loss of balance.

Rooting is important in T'ai Chi both to the extent that the efficiency of issuing power is directly related to good rooting, and to the extent that the redirection or neutralization of any incoming force can be effectively thwarted. The martial issue of interfacing with the direct force of another individual aside, good rooting is important because it qualifies our relationship to the earth on which we live. It helps us to feel, and to be, more grounded. This occurs not just within the context of T'ai Chi practice per se, but in a more general sense as we move through our lives on a daily basis. Rooting our bodies in a physical sense can also serve as a model for how we respond to the non-physical negative energy that others might send our way.

> The ability to root our bodies to the earth, as one consequence of our T'ai Chi practice, can so affect the clarity with which we take in and process information from the world around us that it is almost like having an additional sense organ.

ALL POWER COMES FROM THE EARTH

In truth, everything we accomplish as a result of moving our bodies can be traced back to our physical connection to the earth. By way of illustration, (see Figure 4-1) imagine yourself facing a same size partner, both of you suspended in midair by ropes and harnesses. If you were to push against your partner, all things being equal, both of you would move equally away from each other in response to the force of your push. Neither of you would be able to push to advantage over the other while suspended. It is only when we have something to push or pull against that we are able to issue force more in one direction than any other (see Figure 4-2). This is because every force has a reaction or bounce back force that serves as an impetus for all movement. Without bounce back force we would not have echoes, neither would there be basketball, baseball, or soccer, nor even percussive music.

STRESS CAN UNROOT YOU

Developing a good root can, as do many of the other aspects of T'ai Chi proficiency, present its own unique set of challenges. One of the most obvious hurdles to be overcome is the natural tendency to store stress (See Chapter on Stress) in the upper regions of the body, thus raising one's center of balance. This again is because we live in a very fast paced and cerebral culture, versus one that is slower and more deliberate in its connection to the earth. In making the effort to learn to relax and sink down to get a root, you may find, just as was the case in the earlier chapter on relinquishing stress, that your efforts to become proficient at T'ai Chi put you at odds with some aspects of your chosen lifestyle.

Fairly benign examples of this might include slouching while you drive, chatting on the telephone while securing it to your ear with your shoulder, or unilateral exercise or fitness regimes that emphasize the use of one side of the body, more or less, to the exclusion of the other. Deeper issues more reflective of who you are, versus what you do, will naturally be ingrained and more challenging to overcome. Examples of this might include a tendency to store unresolved anger in your shoulders or upper back, or a disintegrated cerebral orientation that keeps you stuck in your head while being out of touch with your feelings, or perhaps an impatient and fast paced (disproportionately goal oriented) lifestyle. The more deeply entrenched that those issues

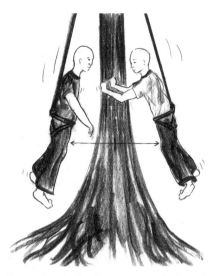

Figure 4-1. Both subjects are repelled equally away from the center by a push in mid-air.

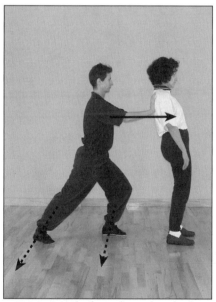

Figure 4-2. The force directed out by the pusher (solid arrow) is only made possible by an equal and opposite force down to the earth (broken line).

disconnecting you from yourself and the earth are, the more time, patience, and outside intervention will be required to implement lasting change.

Lifestyles today all too often, can leave us feeling as if our lives are not fully our own. Commuting in urban traffic, rushing to meet deadlines, or scrambling to see that our kids are fed when we have forgotten to do the shopping or are late for work, are all examples of ways that life can feel a bit much to handle. For many people, when life feels out of hand the natural tendency, though not the healthiest, is to tighten up versus lighten up, and retreat or retrench a bit as the body/mind manifests its natural coping mechanism, the internalization of stress and tension.

You will recall how we discussed in the earlier chapter on stress that the best way to begin to deal with the effects of stress is by becoming more mindful of your own internal processes. By becoming more self-aware, you are taking those first steps necessary to relinquish, or to surrender, stress and tension from the body/mind. Enhanced self-awareness is the first step in learning to relax so that you can acquire a T'ai Chi root. If you have not yet read or tried for yourself the two exercises, "Identifying Stress and Tension Held in the Body," and "Conscious Abdominal Breathing," described in the earlier chapter on Stress, now would be a good time to go back and read or review those sections.

GET A ROOT, GET A LIFE

Following are some exercises that you can experiment with on your own, or in collaboration with a partner, to develop and improve your root. First though, I want to share an anecdote to illustrate what can happen when you try to root without first learning to relax.

Back in the mid 1980's, I was actively involved in a large T'ai Chi/Ch'i Kung organization. Each summer I sat on the examination board to certify new instructors in both T'ai Chi and Iron Shirt Ch'i Kung, two related internal disciplines, each emphasizing rooting skills in their own way. One of the ways we examiners measured the instructor candidates' skills was by pushing them from various angles as they held certain postures, this to assess their ability to both recognize and then redirect an incoming force through their bodies and down to the earth. I recall one morning in particular as I watched several hopefuls practicing with each other in preparation for their test. One woman was sinking overly low in her stance, (see Figures 4-3a, b) clearly mistaking muscle strength for body structure. Whenever someone pushed against her, she responded by pushing back, which only served to reinforce her mistake, as she could not very well be re-channeling force through her body while she was pushing back against that same force. As long as she was resisting and fighting back, there was very little incentive let alone opportunity for her to be guided by a mindful or conscious awareness of what was not working. In other words, she could not fight back while at the same time surrendering to trust her body's inner structure.

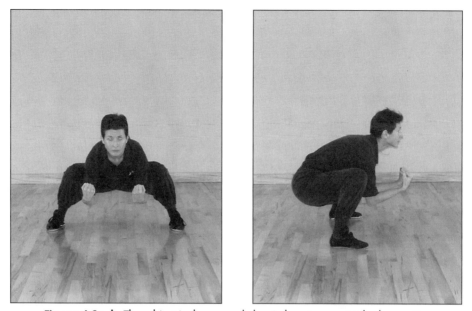

Figures 4-3a, b. The subject is shown overly low in her stance, mistakenly equating depth of stance with quality of rooting.

INVEST IN LOSS

In T'ai Chi we have a saying: "Invest in Loss." This, like most other such profundities, can be understood and applied variably, according to circumstances. In her case, this woman needed to just relax and trust her body's structure to absorb and process the incoming force. As she had no preexisting model, this seemed an unlikely accomplishment. So I walked over and offered her some coaching assistance, just as I do here for you with the following procedures as models.

In the case of this woman, I physically readjusted her posture, straightening her up a bit so that she was less blatantly reliant on muscular force. I placed my hands on her shoulder and hip in preparation to push her, as had her earlier partner. Immediately on feeling my touch, she sank back down and tensed her muscles. I gently coaxed her to relax, breathe, and trust her structure before commencing with any push. Once she was able to let go and relax a bit, I began to push very softly and very slowly in a manner designed not to uproot her, but rather to help her to feel the current of force through her body and down to the earth (see Figures 4-4a, b). Her posture held accordingly, and she expressed pleasant surprise that the intent of my push had so clearly been one of advocacy rather than one of challenge. This idea of being your partner's advocate, is an important point to remember once you get to the two-person practice phase in the following exercises.

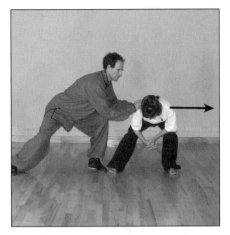

Figure 4-4a. Here the beginner subject cannot hold her root. By pushing across and out, versus across and down, the pusher will merely foster frustration and reinforce bad habits in his beginner subject.

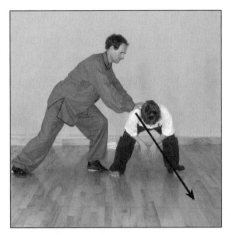

Figure 4-4b. Here, the pusher directs his push "cooperatively" across and down through the subject, aiming to the earth so that she is encouraged to feel a correct skeletal alignment.

STATIONARY SOLO PRACTICE

An effective way for you to work on developing your root, in the absence of a practice partner, is to employ visualization techniques. Let me emphasize that visualization in this context is active versus passive. The key is to practice your visualization while you are engaging your body, rather than practice it as a separate mind-only discipline. Visualization, in this manner, becomes a means by which you can both engage and exploit the body/mind's relaxation response in order to lower your physical and energetic center of balance. One traditional visualization that has proven

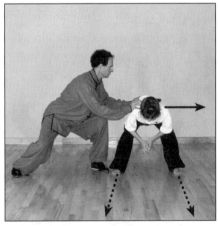

Figure 4-4c. Eventually, the person being pushed will be able to redirect even an "uncooperative" push (solid line) through to the earth (broken line).

useful in helping students to get their root, has been to liken one's proper T'ai Chi posture to a large sturdy tree rooted deeply into the earth (see Figure 4-5). Indeed, many books on T'ai Chi depict illustrations of T'ai Chi'ers with roots extending from their feet down into the earth. Teachers often guide their students helping them to visualize their hands and fingers as soft and supple as leaves in a gentle breeze, their torsos more solid yet still flexible like an oaken trunk, and their feet like roots sending rootlets downwards. This visualization has helped innumerable students get that feeling of being more solidly connected to the earth.

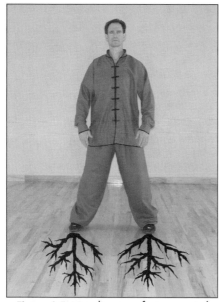

Figure 4-5. Visualize your feet connected down to the earth as roots of a tree.

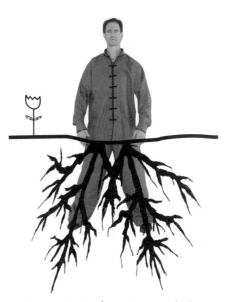

Figure 4-6. Even better, imagine the legs themselves as taproots secured firmly into the earth.

Some time back I heard a much-improved version of this scenario. In sharing this new technique I want to credit an individual whom I regard as a T'ai Chi visionary. Master Wei Lun Huang is the man responsible for introducing me to, among many other things, this conceptual variant. Whereas in the former visualization the idea was to feel yourself rooted to the earth from your feet downwards, in Master Huang's version you will imagine yourself connected from the waist down. Rather than visualizing roots extending down from the bottoms of your feet, you will feel that your legs themselves are long taproots extending downwards from the torso (see Figure 4-6). Imagine that you have stepped down into a hole that is waist deep. Now that you are standing in that hole, slowly backfill it as you hold your stance so that once the hole has been filled you are below ground from the waist down. Your legs are now your roots. As you picture this scenario, it is easy to see and feel how much more firmly you will be anchored in your connection to the earth than if you were merely standing atop it. Nobody will be able to push you off from this position. It would be like trying to push the earth.

Though this and the following techniques are clearly intended to enhance the quality of your T'ai Chi, the principles of rooting and structure are universal and as such, are applicable to a wide range of other disciplines, including sports and fitness. While writing this chapter on rooting I sent one of my editors an excerpt for review, which included the preceding visualization exercise. She wrote back with her usual professional critique, but included the following personal account describing how she had tried to use the visualization described for an activity other than T'ai Chi:

I was struck by how much of what you said is similar to what I've heard from my yoga teachers as to grounding and being connected to the earth. Given those similarities, I thought that I would apply the technique described to the asanas that I practice, beginning with a basic mountain pose and then working into the balancing poses. What a tremendous difference that visualization made. I've never felt so steady, balanced or rooted while maintaining flexibility and the ability to flow into and out of the poses. There has always been one asana that gave me difficulty — half moon pose — where you balance on one foot and one hand while raising the opposite foot and hand. Previously, I could get into this pose but could not hold it well at all, not until I visualized the grounded leg and arm as being buried into the earth. Presto — stillness, balance, calm and a much stronger sensation of energy flow than I'd experienced before. If I never learn another thing from you, I will be grateful. With this you have revolutionized my practice."

As you can see from her account, this particular visualization can be quite powerful in influencing the way we perceive and work with our bodies. Initially, you should limit your work with either of these visualization scenarios to a stationary mode, preferably the basic T'ai Chi opening stance (see Figure 4-7). Later, once you feel ready, you can vary your choice of stance or position as you prefer.

PUSHING WITHOUT PUSHING

Working in collaboration with a partner is one of the best ways to learn practical rooting skills, both as a pusher, and as a pushee. Understand however, that if the partner who is doing the pushing always tries to uproot the pushee, what will usually ensue for the person being pushed is either a feeling of tension or one of competition, either with the pusher or with himself. In this case you may end up like the woman described earlier, overly focused on the goal, and unable to trust your own process. By approaching this exercise with your partner in a collaborative fashion, by *pushing without pushing*, the possible source of tension/competition never materializes.

> It is always easier to trust that you can accomplish a given task or skill when there is no impending opportunity to fail.

The following exercise will demonstrate how this works.

STATIONARY PRACTICE WITH A PARTNER

Once your partner is in position to be pushed (any T'ai Chi posture can be adapted to this exercise) and signals that she is ready, place your hands on her as if to push. At first though, instead of pushing, simply maintain a firm but gentle contact, assuring your partner verbally that you will hold this touch but not push her with it for the time being. Encourage her to visualize a line of energy or force

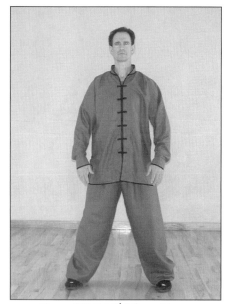

Figure 4-7. Tai Chi Open Stance

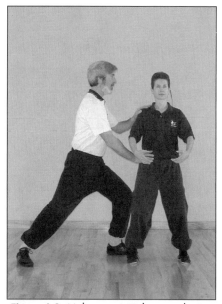

Figure 4-8. Make your initial contact by just touching, without pushing, to help your subject relax. In this way she can come to feel, and trust, her own structure.

from your touch point(s) down through her skeletal structure to the opposite foot and on into the earth (see Figure 4-8). Without the distraction of an anticipated push your partner should be better able to relax and to trust that her structure will act simply as a conduit for the force of your push once it comes. When you do begin to push, be sure to direct your force downward, through her skeletal structure toward the feet, rather than across the body (see Figures 4-9a, b). At first this may seem as if it makes the task for the person being pushed ridiculously simple, but it will reinforce in your partner's body/mind both how her body can function as a conduit for incoming force, and also that the process is the goal. It also will provide your partner an encouraging sense of *can-do* which keeps the practice fun as well as productive. Newer students are much more likely to feel encouraged in continuing their practice by their accomplishments rather than by their failures, so remember to start out pushing to your partner's strengths.

With the improvement in skill level that is bound to result from continued practice, you can raise the angle of your push and increase your pushing force gradually as the pushee becomes increasingly confident in her ability to redirect incoming force through the body and down to the earth (see Figure 4-9c). Remember to keep it simple at first. It is better to progress slowly than to risk falling back into old patterns. Eventually you can vary the angle of the push, or the amount of force applied, keeping in mind that this is a learning exercise not a contest. Over time you can experiment with other variations to this practice. One

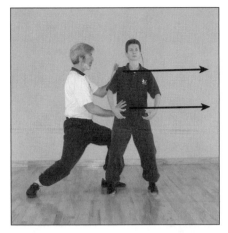

Figure 4-9a. In this photo the pusher directs his force incorrectly across and up, in a manner designed to uproot the subject. If the subject is new at this practice she will neither hold her root, nor improve her level of skill.

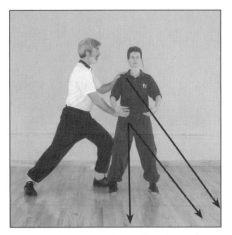

Figure 4-9b. Here the pusher directs his force deliberately down through the subject's skeletal frame so she can feel the transfer of force through her body to the earth.

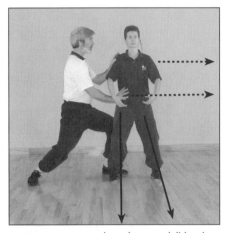

Figure 4-9c. As the subject1s skill level improves, the pusher can raise the pushing angle in order to challenge the subject's ability to redirect an incoming force down to the earth.

variation is to push first with one hand and then smoothly transition to push with the other hand that is located elsewhere on your partner's body. In this manner your partner can begin to learn to adapt his response to pushes from different angles. Be sure to avoid any fast or jerky moves that are more likely to call into play the body/mind's natural response of tightening or retrenching in response to real or perceived danger. The idea here is to stay relaxed and trust your connection to the earth. See Figures 4-10 through 4-15 for examples of how you might try pushing.

NON-PHYSICAL BENEFITS OF ROOTING: EMOTIONAL ROOTING

If you have ever had the experience of being caught off guard by someone's unexpected negativity—a remark, or a malevolent glare, or just a threatening presence—you are a candidate for rooting of a different sort. The energy of negative thought is very similar to physical energy in terms of its inertia. Inertia is the tendency for any energy to remain unchanged in its motion or state unless and until acted upon by another force. It is really up to you whether or not you want to be

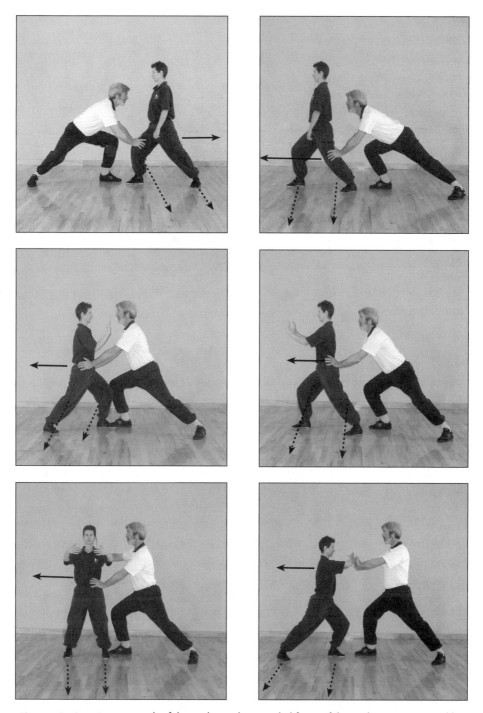

Figures 4-10 to 4-15. In each of these photos the intended force of the pusher is represented by the solid arrow. The subject's redirection of that force is represented by the broken arrow.

that other force that diverts and "catches" someone else's incoming garbage energy. In order to avoid being the brunt of other peoples' verbal abuse or mal-intent, the very same principles that allow you to act as a simple conduit for physical force can be employed here. This is not to say that no one will ever pose a genuine threat, nor is it to say that emotional rooting will render you oblivious to any threat that may require your full or immediate attention. What emotional rooting can do, is help you avoid getting stuck with the stress-causing emo-

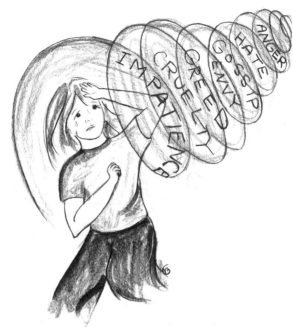

Figure 4-16a. Getting stuck with bad energy.

tions that others may direct your way. The world is full of negative energy, that is to say there is as much potential negative energy as there is positive. You have it within your power to make a choice as to whether or not, and in what manner, you perceive and receive whatever comes your way. There is no special complicated trick to this. If you have managed to grasp the principles of rooting discussed earlier in this chapter, the ability to parry or root negativity down through to the earth will likely present itself as a natural by-product of your T'ai Chi body/mind rooting practices. Just be sure to remember that the determining variable in successfully addressing such energies is the clarity of your attention/intention.

In the same manner that stress embedded in the body can raise your body's center of balance to prevent a stable connection to the earth, unresolved emotional garbage can be a magnet for more of the same. This leaves one increasingly vulnerable to the effects of emotional or psychic assault. As you become better able to resolve and/or relinquish such outstanding issues as stress and anxiety (through T'ai Chi or other adjunctive therapies), you will naturally be less prone to attracting negativity.

To get a sense of how this might work for you, imagine that your body is rooted into the earth like a lightning rod. Now simply imagine another person, someone lacking your skill in dealing with negative energy, saying something angry or hurtful to you. Rather than absorbing this into your consciousness, visualize it passing through your body harmlessly down to the earth (see Figures 4-16a, b). That's all there is to it! It is just like rooting your body physically. Of course I don't mean to be overly simplistic. Sometimes people who are close to us really know how to push our buttons, and so you may have to attend mindfully, noticing for any "flaws" in your non-physical structure. This can help you learn more about yourself. You will need to practice this in order to achieve a level of proficiency, but as you improve you will find yourself naturally less susceptible to the distraction of emotional assault.

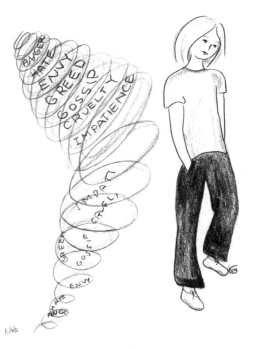

Figure 4-16b. Redirecting bad energy down to the earth.

Notwithstanding the above, there are times when the negative energies people send us, or the critical things they have to say, may be just what we really need, however unpleasant they may feel at the time. Understand that emotional rooting is not intended to be used as a form of blanket denial, or as a facade to avoid your personal accountabilities. You must learn how to distinguish between the good negative and the bad negative and use your skills accordingly.

CONCLUSION

Rooting is just one of the many valuable skills T'ai Chi has to offer. In truth, none of the skills inherent in T'ai Chi are entirely separate from any others. The implications of rooting are far-reaching in their potential to improve the quality of our lives on many levels. Rooting in its simplest manifestation, connects us to our earth, but also serves as a model as well as a means by which we can interact more favorably with a wide range of outside forces. Take this to heart in your own practice. (And may the force move through you.)

In the next chapter we will explore the implications of force from a somewhat different perspective.

Note: For more skilled practitioners, advanced rooting practices are covered in Chapter 12.

THINGS TO REMEMBER:

- Rooting qualifies our relationship to the earth we live on.
- Rooting can reduce falls and injuries in the elderly.
- Enhanced self-awareness is the first step in relaxing and rooting.
- The best way to minimize stress is by remaining mindful of your internal process.
- When practicing rooting with a partner work from advocacy rather than challenge.
- Practice trusting yourself when there is no impending opportunity to fail.
- You always have it within your power to make a choice.

CHAPTER 5

T'ai Chi as an Exercise in Displacement

The generals have a saying:
"Rather than make the first move it is better to wait and see.
Rather than advance an inch it is better to retreat a yard."
This is called going forward without advancing, pushing back with-
out using weapons. When two great forces oppose each other the
victory will go to the one that knows how to yield."
—Tao Te Ching *(Chapter 69)*

WHERE WE STAND IN THE TAO

I remember a time quite a bit earlier in my career when I was between schools of my own. I had recently moved back to the suburban Boston area from a teaching stint elsewhere, and had reconnected with a number of my former students, two of whom had a large coastal estate that they generously made available to me for teaching purposes. Out in the middle of their yard overlooking the ocean was a trellised area large enough within for the practice of T'ai Chi. It was a peaceful little place, and a favorite spot of mine with an abundance of happy chirping birds. I always made a point to arrive early enough before my classes began, to indulge myself some mindful practice time alone amidst the bird songs. I remember not wanting to disturb the *wa* of this little den. And so, I bore this in mind as my moves unfolded one into another. Any jerkiness or unnatural quality to my movement tended to spook my bird friends, thus I sought to remain inconspicuous in my practice. I tried to blend into the Tao, to become just another part of the natural setting. At a later time, removed from that setting, I reflected on T'ai Chi as one small piece of a greater whole, and this reflection afforded me a deeper understanding of T'ai Chi's place amongst the 10,000 things.

CONSEQUENCES, TANGIBLE AND OTHERWISE

One of the areas where western science has flirted with Taoist concepts is in the realm of Chaos Theory.[1] Inherent in this theory is the idea, for example, that a butterfly fluttering its wings in Nepal can affect weather patterns in the eastern U.S. (Curiously, this is called the Butterfly Theory.) The basic premise of Chaos

Theory is that all things are connected in ways that we cannot begin to explain and yet there are no coincidences in life or in nature. The corollary to this is that nothing of consequence is without consequence. Everything has causes and effects that in turn result in more causes and effects. Nothing in nature can be truly presumed to be the result of a single cause or assigned a single effect. Even in western science there is a phenomenon recognized as the *experimenter effect* in which the true objectivity of any experiment is always in question because of the very presence or involvement of those conducting it. No matter how smart we think we are we can never understand anything absolutely. Consequently, our best understanding of anything must always be qualified by relativism.

The Taoist explanation of this phenomenon would be that the butterfly's wings manifest an action (Yang), inevitably resulting in consequences (Yin), which in turn produce other actions, and so on. Yin and Yang thus perpetuate each other. Ebb and flow alone are universal constants. Excepting these, the only absolute is the absence of anything absolute.

Neither can our experience of the T'ai Chi form practice be absolute or finite. Not unless we (self) limit the parameters of our capacity for thought and awareness, but that would be antithetical to T'ai Chi. Rather, we as T'ai Chi players strive to open ourselves to the unknown possibilities in the realization that T'ai Chi is one small but influential part of a greater whole.

One way we can do this is by thinking of T'ai Chi as an exercise in displacement. Because we are so accustomed to moving on this earth, we tend never to think what it is we are moving through, but it is certainly not a void. Hypothetically, if you tried to practice your form while submersed to your neck in thick honey, or even just under water in a pool, your experience would be quite different from that of practicing on dry land. Yet even on dry land, when you change your position to move through the air across the earth's surface, you are not just moving through the air, you are displacing it. Two different matters cannot occupy the same space at the same time. The implication of your movement is that in changing any position you must simultaneously move something else. Whenever you move something else, it will move something else, and that will move something else, and so on, in a rippling effect forever outward. Thus by moving, like the butterfly fluttering its wings, you create a disturbance in the Tao, the ultimate consequences of which one can only begin to imagine. Nothing of consequence is without consequence, and indeed everything is of consequence.

ON A LARGER SCALE

If we take a closer look at this concept of displacement from the perspective of scale, you will see for example, that a pebble tossed into a quiet pool will cause an outward rippling effect, but not to the same extent as a larger rock thrown into the same pool (see Figures 5-1a, b). Here I will direct your attention to one of the important skills that T'ai Chi teaches, *Ting Jing*, or listening skill (See Glossary).

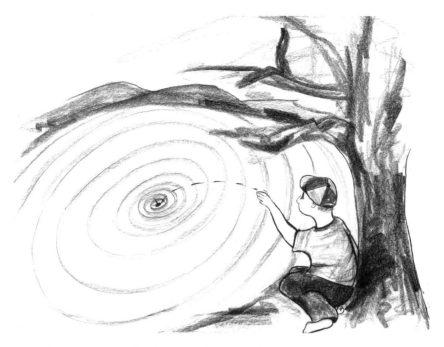

Figure 5-1a. A small pebble tossed into a pool creates a minor disturbance...

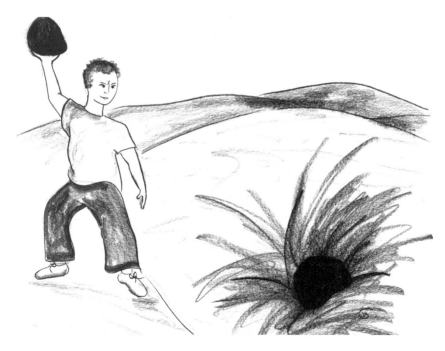

Figure 5-1b. ...while a larger rock makes a big splash.

This skill is generally called to mind in the context of Pushing Hands practice where it is important to listen to, or to perceive, an opponent's intention via the sensitivity of one's touch (see Figure 5-2). By so listening, one can remain sensitive to any impending danger and avoid being caught off guard. That same sensitivity can be used to avoid compromising (by telegraphing) one's own best interests in initiating any action, as well as in responding to the actions of others. When you learn to listen, particularly in regard to the anticipated consequences of your own actions, you are more likely to conduct your behavior conscientiously

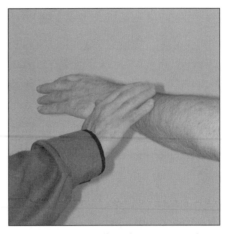

Figure 5-2. A soft and sensitive touch enables one to develop Ting Jing listening skill.

and in harmony with the Tao. I believe this skill has implications on a grander scale as well. Today the very health of our planet Earth is in jeopardy because it has been poorly stewarded by individuals who have neglected to listen (insufficient Yin), and have thus failed to perceive the fuller impact of what amounts to their having thrown too many rocks into the pool (excess Yang). Our world today is rife with the consequences of poorly thought out actions. All forms of pollution such as nuclear/biological threat, iatrogenic medical complications, consumer waste, over population/crowding, (this is the short list), are consequences of a population having acted without listening or anticipating.

Given the potential magnitude of our initiative in any action, it behooves us to pay close attention to those actions lest we miss something important or misstep along the way.

> What I mean to say is that in committing ourselves to a practice of T'ai Chi, in quest of mindful martial excellence, we have by extension committed ourselves to becoming better human beings.

Just as the energetic effects of our own actions ripple out far and wide, so I believe do the effects of our intentions, our feelings, and the choices we make in life. Becoming a better human being carries something of a mandate to leave the world a better place for its having hosted our visits. We as T'ai Chi practitioners are gifted with a unique opportunity. Our commitment to T'ai Chi assigns us a role as self-appointed stewards of the world we live in. Accepting this role, we agree to listen carefully, so as to pursue the right course of action or inaction as the case may be, in order to remain in harmony with the Tao (Yin and Yang in balance). This can manifest on a variable scale. It can be as involved as working actively for global change in some form or another, or it can simply be a quietly held conviction that you are a small but integral part of a larger whole. Remember, nothing is so insignificant as to be without significance.

One of the things T'ai Chi has taught me is that life is a celebration, an ongoing blessed event. This powerful awareness commands my attention and reminds me to move mindfully, there being no time for mindlessness. In recalling that our topic here is one of displacement, I would add that even in the fourth dimension, the dimension of time, displacement plays a critical role. As each new moment unfolds, it does so at the expense of the moment at hand. And just as no thought, belief, or action can be presumed to be without consequence, every moment is unique and irreplaceable and therefore precious.

DISPLACEMENT EXERCISE

As a practical matter, in regards to your own practice, you can experiment with the following T'ai Chi exercise to get a sense of how this concept of displacement can be of tangible relevance to you.

As you stand in preparation to begin your form practice imagine the air around you has taken on a consistency that is visually discernible as would be smoke or steam. If, for example, you were to swing your arms in such a smoke filled room, your arm movements would displace air and the resultant air currents would cause the smoke to swirl about (see Figure 5-3). Alternately, imagine moving your arms slowly yet so effortlessly as to cause little or no disturbance in the smoke (see Figure 5-4). Now as you actually embark on your practice, try to keep your movements as discreet as possible. The movements need not be small, but you will need to keep them slow, smooth, and unobtrusive in order to minimize any disturbance they might otherwise cause by stirring the air. Conscientiously, match your movements to your breath and use your *Ting Jing* listening skill to try to feel, really feel, exactly what is displaced with each movement or shift of any part of your body. This may prove to be more difficult than you might at first imagine. Allow each move to realize its full range, and yet, keep it contained within the limits of its design. By practicing in this way, your movements will cause minimal disturbance in the imaginary atmosphere around you, and you will enhance your ability for sensitivity to even the smallest force, in this case, the mere resistance of the air around you.

If you are sensitive enough to recognize how technique or poor posture may be causing you to unnecessarily disrupt air currents, this practice will also afford you insights as to where your form may be remiss in terms of extraneous movement. Always employ the least amount of movement necessary, and remain soft so as to adhere to the T'ai Chi principle of using a minimum force or effort to realize any given action. Of course your T'ai Chi is only valuable to the extent that you can apply it to the rest of your life. As you move through your day, try to bear in

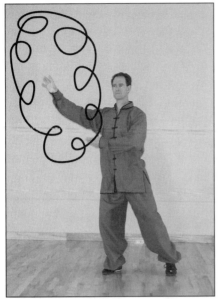

Figure 5-3. Unwieldy, fast, or jerky movements create a disturbance in the Tao.

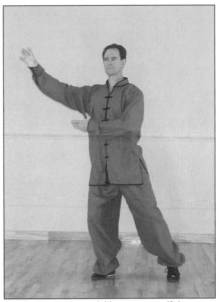

Figure 5-4. Slow, deliberate, mindful movements keep one in harmony with the Tao.

mind the principles of displacement in your interactions with others and the impact of these principles on the decisions you make. (See Appendix A and B for T'ai Chi Principles.)

EMOTIONAL DISPLACEMENT

According to TCM (traditional Chinese medicine), the body's organ systems have the capacity to house various emotional energies. Referring to the chart below, one can see for example that the liver can store, and serve as a venue for the expression of anger or, conversely, kindness.

As a practical matter these dual emotions resident to any particular organ are, when in a state of excess, functionally incompatible. They will in fact serve to displace each other because too much of one means too little of the other. In other words, for someone who is very angry either acutely or as part of his or her core

Lungs:	Grief/melancholy or Courage/integrity
Kidneys:	Fear or Gentleness
Liver:	Anger/rage or Kindness
Heart:	Cruelty/impatience or Joy/respect
Spleen:	Worry/neurosis or Balance/fairness/harmony

Figure 5-5. Five Elements emotional correspondences.

personality, the virtue of kindness will be less accessible. Someone who is afraid or who lives in fear will not be able to realize his or her full potential for gentleness. Conversely, the person who is naturally balanced will be less prone to neurosis, and the person for whom joy and respect are prominent features will be less susceptible to impatience and cruelty.

In practicing T'ai Chi we are concerned with ourselves as whole beings, consequently we must take into account the effects that our emotional state bears upon us. There are no emotions that are innately bad, but all emotions must be held in a relative balance. There are adjunctive meditation/Ch'i Kung practices premised specifically on the correlation's outlined above, their goal being to restore harmony by (re)balancing the emotions. Any detailed discussion of such practices is beyond the scope of this book. However you may bear in mind that within this concept of displacement and cause and effect, energies of the emotional, cognitive, or spiritual realm are every bit as significant as the more obvious physical manifestations.

Two volumes that I would recommend for practical reference on the subject of emotional energy and the Tao are, *Taoist Ways to Transform Stress Into Vitality* and *Fusion of the Five Elements I,*[2] available at your bookstore or through the Healing Tao Press.

DISPLACEMENT AND APPLICATION

Regarding the implication of displacement to application (application being that aspect of T'ai Chi that deals with the use of its techniques in actual combat situations), it bears repeating that two different matters cannot simultaneously occupy the same time and space. As obvious as this may seem, it is an important yet elusive concept to exploit functionally for martial purposes. Displacement is the Yang essence of using your force to encroach on the force or space of an opponent. Any initiating attempt you make, applying your T'ai Chi to strike, redirect, uproot, or otherwise render your opponent harmless, will necessarily entail displacement in one form or another. By remaining cognizant of the principles of displacement, versus simply executing a technique, you will find yourself better equipped to call on your skills in adapting to the demands of variable circumstances.

ENVELOPING AS A COROLLARY TO DISPLACEMENT

In keeping with the ever pervasive concept of reciprocal duality (there is no Yin without Yang), I would emphasize that displacement also has its own corollary, that of *envelopment*. Whatever displaces something else must necessarily be enveloped in the process. For example, if you simply extend your arm and fist it will displace air and it will simultaneously be enveloped by the air around. For a more tangible experience of this you might try submersing your arm and fist into a tub of water. As your fist submerges displacing water, it will naturally be enveloped by the water is has displaced.

Envelopment can be managed to a relative degree when you are on the receiving end of another's force. The relative variable in this case is your ability to "yield". If in responding to the force of another you fail to yield, or you envelop to only a small degree, you may be displaced to a large degree (ouch!) (see Figure 5-6). But if you are able to yield and envelop to a larger degree, you will control your opponent and not be displaced by his or her force. Thus, how proficiently you negotiate the meeting of these two forces, the seeking-displacement force versus the yielding-envelopment force, ultimately will determine whether you are the victor or the vanquished in any meeting of two opposing forces.

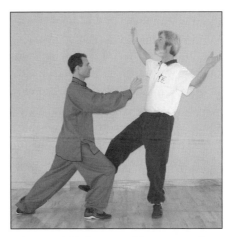

Figure 5-6. Failure to yield to or neutralize an incoming force results in the subject being displaced by that force.

HOW TO ENVELOP AN INCOMING FORCE

Regardless of whether the forces are physical, spiritual, cognitive, or emotional, the same model applies. Let us recall the earlier chart on Five Element Emotional Correlations while imagining that someone approaches you with a powerful feeling of anger (Yang and displacing). If you were to reciprocate with an equally powerful anger of your own, the two Yang forces would collide and remain in unresolved flux. They would remain in a state of conflict and imbalance, until some equally powerful Yin influence presented itself to reestablish a state of balance i.e., exhaustion or capitulation. Of course you can always simply deflect an anger, or refuse to acknowledge it, but the energy is still there, unresolved and potentially threatening.

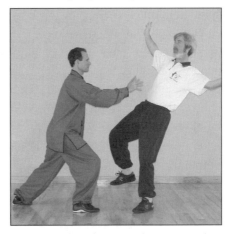

Figure 5-7. When two otherwise equal forces collide, the force stemming from the better root will prevail to displace the less rooted force.

The best solution will probably be to begin by employing a variant of the aforementioned *Ting Jing* listening skill. (Remember, to "listen" in this context simply means to perceive what needs to be perceived.) By perceiving what it is that motivates the other person's anger, you may be better able to anticipate just how you may be in jeopardy. You may realize what it is about you that stands to be displaced (is this other person trying to incite your anger, your submission, your fear, etc.?). By perceiving more clearly what motivates an incoming force, you will be better equipped to yield to and envelop this force. You may determine that kindness, as the complement to anger, is the best way to envelop this force in a

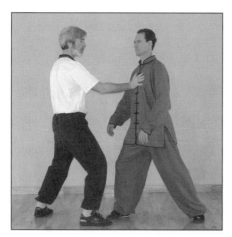 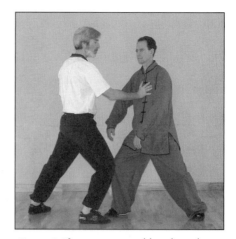

Figure 5-8a. When confronted with a force...

Figure 5-8b. ...you can yield and envelop it in order to neutralize its potential.

way that keeps you intact while bringing both parties to a state of resolution and balance. Or having assessed the situation (meaning you have enveloped it, or taken it in), you can now act in any other appropriate manner. The important point here is that by somehow enveloping the situation (Yin) you become more fully empowered to respond versus react. By responding instead of reacting you are taking initiative and not simply acquiescing to someone else's force.

A second example of this happens again when you find yourself confronted with someone else's effort to displace you. You can fail to yield (in a sense, the same as resisting or pushing back) (see Figure 5-7) and find yourself pushed back (Yang versus Yang), or you can yield and envelop (Yang into Yin) (see Figures 5-8a, b). As with the emotional example cited above, you can simply deflect the incoming force, leaving the energy unresolved, or you can yield before it in a way that allows you to envelop and remain fully in control (see Figures 5-9a, b). Advanced level T'ai Chi practitioners are often able to negotiate incoming forces in this manner so that their responses (Yin and yielding) appear effortless in restoring balance to an otherwise volatile situation.

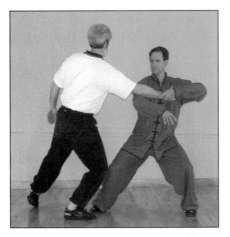

Figure 5-9a. By continuing to yield and envelop...

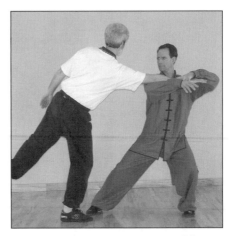

Figure 5-9b. ...you can remain fully in control.

THINGS TO REMEMBER:

- Your best understanding of anything must be qualified by relativism.
- Movement/change will always cause something else to be displaced.
- T'ai Chi'ers must *listen* carefully to know the right course of action or inaction.
- T'ai Chi is only valuable to the extent that you apply it to the rest of your life.
- Whatever displaces something else must be enveloped in the process.
- How proficiently you negotiate displacement vs. envelopment determines your success or failure.

Notes

1. James Gleick. *Chaos, Making a New Science.* 1988.
2. Both books by Mantak Chia.

CHAPTER 6

Form as a Vessel for T'ai Chi Principles

"Many spokes share the wheel's hub;
Yet it is the center hole that makes the wheel useful.
If you form clay into a vessel;
It is the space within that makes it useful.
Cut doors and windows for a room;
And what is not there is what becomes useful.
Therefore, benefit comes from emptiness;
Usefulness from what is not there."
—Tao Te Ching *(Chapter 11)*

LEARN THE PRINCIPLES TO GET THE FORM

When the average person thinks of T'ai Chi, the image that I expect most often comes to mind is one of some person or persons practicing a slow motion T'ai Chi form sequence. This is quite reasonable given T'ai Chi's usual portrayal in the various media. This image is not an entirely incorrect association but it is incomplete. In fact, most people who have not undertaken a formal study of T'ai Chi Ch'uan, and this includes martial artists from other styles, have little idea that there is so much more to T'ai Chi than meets the eye (recall here the metaphor of T'ai Chi as an iceberg, its greater bulk hidden from view). The important principles of T'ai Chi, which serve as a basis for its practice, are generally imperceptible to all but those schooled in their intricacies via lengthy study of the Form. In truth, it is the expression of T'ai Chi's principles that renders the form optimally useful. The form itself is merely a vessel for those principles. [Note: see Appendix A and B for a listing of T'ai Chi Principles.

LEARN THE FORM (WELL) TO GET THE PRINCIPLES

There are many good reasons to practice the T'ai Chi form. In the study of any style, it is the practice of the Form that builds strength, reduces the apparent effects of stress, and teaches balance, fluidity, and more. However, T'ai Chi runs much deeper than the mere series of movements comprising its form. Thus the T'ai Chi form movement sequence should not be misconstrued as representing all that is T'ai Chi. Learning the form well, aside from offering the aforementioned tangible benefits, is also essential in order to learn and embody the full spirit and deeper principles of this ancient discipline. It is the mindful slowness of T'ai Chi that allows us to notice aspects of ourselves not readily apparent at life's usual pace. T'ai Chi does more than merely allow us such notice; it compels it. "Allowing" us and "compelling" us such notice are two significantly different dynamics. Merely "allowing" seems somehow to infer a haphazard or coincidental experience that may or may not present an element of incentive along with the opportunity for such notice. "Compelling" on the other hand, infers a deliberate and unavoidable dynamic which, by design, opens doors into our deeper selves.

In order to gain such access and exploit the full range of benefits that the form has to offer, one needs either unusual insight or a suitable guide. The form itself comes with no assurance that its mere practice will inspire profound insight or illuminate us to T'ai Chi's deeper essences. Open doors, after all, are by themselves only that; we still must choose to pass through those doors. Hypothetically, someone could learn all the movements of a given form, even to the point of performing them well, and still not be doing T'ai Chi, at least not in its more profound sense. I freely admit to this having been so in my own case earlier in my career when, as a young skilled Kung Fu practitioner, I displayed an apparent command of all the superficialities of the T'ai Chi form, but little else. Observers to my practice who knew little or nothing about T'ai Chi were inevitably impressed by my execution of moves, while those more in the know politely withheld comment.

As depicted in chapters elsewhere throughout this book, other qualities requisite to T'ai Chi, besides the mere memorization and execution of the moves, include:

- Rooting to the earth
- Paying attention to Ch'i
- Enhancing one's self-awareness—leading to improved skeletal articulation/alignment, that in turn leads to obtaining more enhanced self-awareness
- Gaining intra-personal insight—hopefully achieving some sense of being part of a larger whole, sociologically as well as universally, and so on, round and round.

T'ai Chi mastery entails an integrative process that transcends the form itself. The "trick" is to somehow "break through" from T'ai Chi as a mere superficial exercise regime, to develop a practical understanding of how these principles and essences can work for you. Once you do that you will be at a point where you can navigate your own course. Until you reach that point, it bears repeating, that the best way to get there is by practicing your form often, and under the guidance of a knowledgeable teacher.

FORM VERSUS NO-FORM

You need the Form in order to get the principles via direct experience. Conveniently inherent in the form is the means for accomplishing just that. But only if you know how to decipher T'ai Chi's "code" will you be able to distill its subtler essences. When all is said and done, it is our mastery of those essences, the embodiment of T'ai Chi's age-old principles, which determines the quality of our practice. I will even go so far as to say paradoxically, that the T'ai Chi form itself, though initially requisite, is ultimately superfluous. This is bound to raise the hackles of some T'ai Chi purists, but the fact remains that there are many different styles of T'ai Chi, each with their own form or forms. It stands to reason that if there were only one right way to do T'ai Chi then there would only be one form or one style necessary or even possible to express that one right way and any other approach would either be redundant or wrong. As it is, there are different styles, with different forms, all of which apparently have withstood the test of time on their own merits. Thus the benefits of T'ai Chi must not be inherent in the moves of any particular form per se, but rather in one's interpretation and expression, through the form, of the underlying principles. You do need the form in order to fully comprehend and experience the principles, but the principles must be understood first, prior to relative mastery, just as an art student needs to learn how to mix paint before expressing himself through painting. Then, just as mixing paint eventually becomes second nature to the skilled artist, requiring little practice, once you have learned the principles of T'ai Chi the expression of those principles lends itself to almost any context, within or without the form.

Conveniently again, the form is not only the best vehicle for *learning* the principles, it also remains the ideal venue for *expressing* those principles. Through it one can extract the myriad benefits that T'ai Chi has to offer and apply those benefits in life outside of T'ai Chi class or form practice. This raises some interesting questions. Once an advanced level has been reached and the form has been mastered so that its benefits permeate one's life, does one then no longer need to practice in order to continue to derive benefit? Should one then discard or neglect the form? Is T'ai Chi mastery akin to earning a doctorate, suggesting perhaps that one has gained the requisite bulk of knowledge to remain proficient? I think not. Rather it is just the opposite. None of life's lessons are any more static than we are as individuals. Just because we may be in a better place now than where we were previously does not mean we neither have anything more to learn nor room for further personal growth.

Is asking whether or not we should continue to practice once relative mastery has been achieved a silly question? Again, I think not. The question really brings to the forefront the contrast between Tai Chi as a personal learning process and other conventional learning venues; the likes of which many of us experienced as we were growing up. In our Western culture, education is often approached or presented in a linear fashion. From grade school on, students typically undertake studies of interest (or obligation) to be followed through step by step to a logical conclusion, at which point attention is simply refocused elsewhere. In my opinion, *linear learning* is overly focused on the goal rather than the process. This unfortunately creates a tendency toward linear thinking, which limits one's creative possibilities. Happily, T'ai Chi espouses a different paradigm, one in which the process of learning remains a goal unto itself. Thus the T'ai Chi form remains an ideal environment in which to reinforce our growth as an ongoing process and its continued practice is an opportunity to celebrate all that we have already learned.

FORM WITHOUT STRUCTURE

I had an experience some years back with a student who enrolled in my class after having taken some seminars with Al Chung-liang Huang at the Esalon Institute in Big Sur. Al Huang, who eschews the title of Master, wrote a delightful book on T'ai Chi back in 1973 entitled *Embrace Tiger Return to Mountain*, in which he refreshingly espoused the benefits of T'ai Chi as a model for living without stricture. No reflection, I am sure, on Al Huang, but this woman seemed to have (mis)interpreted his teachings to mean that there was *never* any need for structure. She made the mistake of doing what followers often do, which is to hear one thing and somehow manage to translate it as something else in reflection of her own agenda.

STRUCTURE OR STRICTURE

Once enrolled in my class, she was all over the place swinging her arms as if dancing to imaginary music (fine at home, perhaps, but not in T'ai Chi class). This woman completely lacked structure, but more significantly, she lacked any desire for structure or willingness to consider its merits. She wanted to be like an abstract artist but she did not want to be bothered with learning how to mix paint before getting to her canvas. Unwilling to be bound in any way by T'ai Chi convention, she made a poor student. She must have thought me a poor teacher as well, because she quickly lost interest in my teaching method which emphasized the importance of structured basics as a foundation for future learning.

One other sad mistake this woman made was to confuse the feeling of being truly free and in the moment with the tendency to indulge her need for immediate gratification. She had an open (though undisciplined) body, but a closed mind.

> Freedom comes from structure, not from abandon. To become skilled at T'ai Chi one must first experience structure. What this woman failed to understand was that one of the eventual results of embodying the principles of T'ai Chi structure is to be able to move in such a manner as to appear to be free of structure. Ultimately, structure has the potential to free us from stricture.

GET YOUR BODY IN THE MOMENT

A recurring theme throughout this book, first mentioned in the Introduction as one of the important benefits that T'ai Chi has to offer, is *being in the moment*. Usually, this quality or state is thought of in the context of one's mind and of one's *awareness* being in the moment. However T'ai Chi, via its emphasis on structure, teaches us the importance of keeping our *bodies* in the moment as well. As challenging as it can be for many people to be mentally in the moment, it is probably easier to be so with our minds than it is with our bodies. When you are paying attention to just your mind, though there may be myriad distractions, there is only one single consciousness of which to keep track. When attending to the body there are dozens of disparate parts, each seemingly having a separate "mind" of its own.

Improper practice habits can preclude one from staying in the moment. Habits such as allowing the body to bounce up at the expense of the root, failing to maintain a continuous flow of force to and from the ground (known as unfolding), or limiting oneself by holding stress or tension anywhere in the body, are just a few examples of ways that the body, in being out of the moment, can interfere with the mind's ability to be truly in the moment. Conversely, when your root remains solid while flowing through all of your moves, and when all of the body parts are connected so as to facilitate an optimally efficient release (or receipt) of power, and when stress and tension have been relinquished freeing the body of its limitations, the mind quite naturally follows suit. One's experience of being in the moment transcends either body or mind to become more fully an experience of the body/mind as an integrative process.

Visiting that place of body/mind integration can be challenging enough, but residing there permanently can be more than challenging, even under the best of circumstances. I recall being on holiday at the beach, completely free of the usual obligations of business and teaching, and thus able to indulge myself more fully in the spontaneity of the moment. One sunny morning I arose to start the day with a round of Ch'i Kung stretching and meditation prior to my morning swim. As I concluded my practice, reflecting back on how wonderful and truly connected it had made me feel, I promptly tripped while pulling on my swimming trunks and fell clumsily to the floor. I felt like a klutz and I remember laughing out loud at myself as I sheepishly realized how my mind, so indulged in the delightful moments of an experience just past, prevented my body from being fully present to the moment at hand.

STRUCTURE BEGETS RESILIENCE

Indeed, T'ai Chi would be of little value if it were to become just one more rigid pattern in your life. Though rigidity and resilience are relative and non-exclusive terms, most of us have in our minds the idea that rigidity infers an unyielding quality, while resilience suggests strength in flexibility. Notwithstanding that, one must experience structure in order to understand structure and thus exploit its benefits without becoming confined within its bounds. Structure within form is what allows for a consistent experience of T'ai Chi principles by insuring that disparate parts of the body remain reliably and manageably connected. This allows for a consistent application of principles, regardless of scale, so that we can readily observe even the biggest principles manifesting in the smallest move, never losing the trees for the forest. Structure is not synonymous with rigidity. For the purposes of T'ai Chi, inherent in its structure is the concept of resilience. It is the resilience, not the rigidity, of the tall oak that allows it to withstand a great wind.

"LIVING" T'AI CHI

It may be very easy to form the impression that T'ai Chi masters engaged in their practice represent some distant and unattainable goal which we can only seek but never achieve. In truth, this is not the case.

> The most highly evolved T'ai Chi masters are those who embody T'ai Chi beyond the limits of the Form itself with the understanding that T'ai Chi is as much the act of living as it is the practice of the Form. Each of us, through the practice of T'ai Chi, has the opportunity to comport ourselves as masters-in-process by **living** T'ai Chi instead of merely **doing** T'ai Chi.

We can expand beyond the normal constraints of physical structure by gaining mastery of our physical structure. This is why we should not limit ourselves by thinking of T'ai Chi as a mere movement or exercise pattern. T'ai Chi, as a vessel for its principles, can be a metaphor for how each of us can come to live our lives in the best way possible.

THINGS TO REMEMBER:

- It is the expression of T'ai Chi's principles that render the form useful.
- T'ai Chi mastery entails an integrative process which transcends the form.
- The form is the best way to learn the principles, and remains the best way to express those principles.
- The T'ai Chi learning process is a goal unto itself.
- Freedom comes from structure rather than from abandon.
- Structure can free us from stricture.
- Structure keeps disparate body parts reliably connected.
- T'ai Chi is as much about the act of living as it is the practice of form.

CHAPTER 7

The Role of Ch'i Kung in Relation to T'ai Chi

*"And the Lord formed man of the dust of the ground,
and breathed into his nostrils the breath of life;
and the man became a living soul."*
Genesis 2:7
   —The Bible, *King James Translation*

AN EXERCISE IN FUTILITY

Back in the late 1970's, when I first developed an awareness of Ch'i Kung as a entity separate from T'ai Chi, I had an experience with my Kung Fu master who offered to teach me a "rare" Ch'i Kung practice. This initial Ch'i Kung learning experience was enlightening, if not disillusioning, in several ways. I had mentioned to my Sifu at the time that I was interested in learning to "work more with my Ch'i". He told me I needed to learn a technique that he would impart to me, implying that this was a special exercise he had never before taught to anyone else. I hungrily and naively accepted his offer.

The directions for practicing this particular Ch'i Kung routine were fairly simple, requiring a mere hour or two of guidance on my teacher's part before I had all the details memorized. However the actual practice proved to be grueling. This memorable technique required me to awaken sufficiently early each morning to complete my practice session prior to sunrise. During practice I was required to balance myself while hopping around atop a half dozen Plum Flower poles (logs of variable heights embedded like tree trunks in my yard, according to a specific pattern), while I contorted my body and employed various breathing methods. Naturally, the requisite postures precluded my looking down at my feet as I hopped about the different levels. No doubt this was one of the more difficult, not to mention dangerous, practices I have ever engaged in. My Sifu had made it clear that I was to do this practice daily. He emphasized further, that if I engaged in sexual relations within two weeks (before or after) of doing the practice, I would die! Suffice it to say, I did not have much of a social life, but I was young and idealistic enough (not to mention a bit of a risk taker at that time of my life) that I stuck it out for several months. During the time that I kept up my practice

I definitely began to experience some strange and powerful physiologic phenomena, unquestionably resulting from my efforts at this practice.

A couple of months into this new training, I arranged to meet with my Sifu over breakfast one morning. I took the opportunity to describe my experiences and to ask him some very pointed questions about how he expected me to benefit from the work he had taught me. In response to my description of the energy phenomena I had been experiencing he merely grunted his approval. Then, he proceeded to assure me the exercises were good for my health (That's it?) and reaffirmed that I would surely die if I had sex. I pressed him for more detailed information only to be told that this exercise was "good for my Ch'i". Despite my continued inquiries, no additional information was to be gained. Considering the sacrifices I was making, his responses did not amount to the quality of information I sought and needed in order to remain inspired to keep up my practice. Shortly thereafter, I left this exercise by the wayside in favor of other less inscrutable and socially alienating work.

My point in sharing this experience is that there are varying degrees of sophistication when it comes to the zillion or so different ways to work with energy. Not everyone who purports to teach Ch'i Kung energy work has a detailed understanding of what they are doing, or why. Sometimes these practices are just "stuff" that got passed down from someone's teacher's teacher, with any comprehensive understanding of the true purpose or value lost along the way. This is just one example of how some teachers can be remiss in providing the information necessary for a given practice to become meaningful and relevant to a student's training in particular and to life in general. It also serves as an example of what can happen when a student follows blindly, imbuing a teacher with more trust and credibility than may be warranted.

WHAT IS CH'I KUNG (QIGONG)?

Strictly speaking, T'ai Chi Ch'uan is, or can be, a form of Ch'i Kung. Speaking more generally, Ch'i Kung practices are regarded as separate adjuncts to the study of T'ai Chi. Simply stated, Ch'i Kung can be any form of body practice, dynamic or static, which incorporates mindful and deliberate attention to both the breath and the movement or manifestation of Ch'i in the body. Any Ch'i Kung practice which serves to open the body, to promote awareness of and insights into body structure, and/or to generate the flow of Ch'i, can prove useful as a companion discipline for aspiring T'ai Chi students hoping to optimize the benefits of their practice.

As noted, T'ai Chi has the potential to fit all aspects of this definition, but whether it actually fulfills this potential depends on how it is presented. I know from my own experience that each of my first two T'ai Chi teachers failed to present T'ai Chi in the context of a Ch'i Kung discipline. Rather it was presented merely as a slow motion movement pattern, ostensibly but inexplicably designed to improve one's Ch'i. As I recall, there was no emphasis whatsoever on the specifics of mindfulness or on the cultivation of Ch'i, other than occasional vague references to T'ai Chi being good for one's health. I can only imagine that these early teachers of mine passed down their T'ai Chi as they themselves were taught.

At the other extreme, a third teacher I worked with was a Tao master whose teachings, though quite esoteric, were generally concise and clear enough for his western students to grasp with minimal difficulty. This Tao master took just the opposite approach of my earlier teachers, requiring a comprehensive course in Taoist energy meditation in order to learn how to move, manage, and store Ch'i energy as an integral component to his T'ai Chi instruction. In this latter case, T'ai Chi was definitely presented as a deliberate form of Ch'i Kung.

THREE DIFFERENT CATEGORIES OF CH'I KUNG

In my understanding there are three general categories encompassing the enormously broad range of Ch'i Kung practices. The first of these, *simple* Ch'i Kung, is non-eclectic, having no requisite spiritual affiliation. This category of Ch'i Kung is understood to reinforce the *Wei Ch'i* function and promote balanced energy overall. It is regarded as "simple" because it does not have a specific or complex pattern of energy movement i.e., intentional directing of Ch'i energy via certain acupuncture meridians. The label "simple" should not be misconstrued to imply that the results of this approach are of any less intrinsic value than other versions. Many Ch'i Kung disciplines (i.e., *I Chin Ching/Muscle Changing Classic,* or various forms of "martial" Ch'i Kung) fall into this category, including T'ai Chi Ch'uan, at least through its intermediate stages. Occasionally, newer students at T'ai Chi will have some experience of feeling energy concomitant to their form practice. It is more likely however that newer students' conscious attention to memorization of the moves will preclude any replicable or comprehensive experience of energy phenomena. Such experiences as these are more apt to occur during intermediate or advanced stages of T'ai Chi practice.

The second category is *formulaic* Ch'i Kung, which often relies on more complex "alchemical" criteria to move Ch'i through the body or its surrounding energy fields in very specific patterns i.e., Microcosmic Orbit, Taoist sexual energy practices, or Kan and Li work. Formulaic Ch'i Kung often has clearly identifiable roots in Taoism or Buddhism.

Finally, there is *medical* Ch'i Kung, encompassing a range of practices that may be prescribed by TCM health practitioners as they pertain to specific health conditions. Because I have not had extensive formal training in TCM, I am less familiar with medical Ch'i Kung. However, I have had quite a varied exposure to simple and alchemical Ch'i Kung practices, and it has been my experience that their sophistication and efficacy can vary widely, according to any number of variables. Sitting or standing Ch'i Kung practices can variably be assigned to any of the noted categories, depending on the nature of the energy work inherent in the practice.

WHY CH'I KUNG AS AN ADJUNCT

In comparison to the two teaching extremes described earlier, I prefer a middle path for my own students. I strongly believe that conscious attention to the breath and to the cultivation of Ch'i are important adjuncts to the basic movement patterns inherent in the different T'ai Chi systems. One of the precepts of Taoist energy practice is "the more you do outside the less happens inside, and the less you do outside, the more happens inside." This is why simple sitting meditation is regarded as such an effective means of generating and cultivating Life Force Energy. If you happen to be a newer student at T'ai Chi, and your body/mind is struggling to recall, the one-hundred plus movements from a typical long form, your attention may be sufficiently externalized so as not to be oriented toward a conscious awareness of what is going on deep within yourself. This is not to say that you will not have Chi. We all have Chi whether we feel it or not. You will however, be less likely to be aware of any confirming experience which entails a feeling of your own energy. This is why I feel deliberate Ch'i Kung practice, as an adjunct to form practice, is an ideal way to begin to get in touch with your energy and to effectively catalyze the growth and maturation process of your T'ai Chi.

DIFFERENT STROKES FOR DIFFERENT FOLKS

The teaching approach I prefer is to include simple Ch'i Kung as an integral part of my T'ai Chi program to the point that it is inseparable and at times indistinguishable from form practice. When students feel ready they can augment their T'ai Chi practice with more comprehensive approaches to personal energy cultivation via sitting meditation practices or formulaic Ch'i Kung routines. The more comprehensive practices do require a commitment of time and some discipline to keep them up, so it makes little sense to require these more advanced energy practices for students who are not ready for that level of work. (Few reasons provide a greater disincentive to continue one's studies than being burdened by information overload.) Teachers often must walk a fine line in determining what is best for any given student in the long run, versus what a student is a capable of over the short term.

One final important variable that must be taken into account is the pre-existing health and energy of the student. I have worked with quite a few students over the years whose health, or unbalanced energy, precluded safe integration into their practice of any but the simplest Ch'i Kung work, i.e., simple abdominal breathing. Students with chemical imbalances or addictive or disordered personalities are particularly at risk. It is critical that the teacher be aware of these factors when deciding how, when, or if to integrate more comprehensive energy work into the student's practice.

TEACHING STYLES CAN VARY

As noted earlier, there are varying levels of sophistication in the knowledge and teaching styles of the many teachers sharing this art. I imagine that there are probably a good number of T'ai Chi teachers whose training has not included the deeper internal components of T'ai Chi Ch'uan, or who for one reason or another, choose not to include that information in their own teachings. Of course, there are populations of students for whom such an (untimely) emphasis might be entirely inappropriate. For example, T'ai Chi has become increasingly popular in senior centers. For many elderly people just learning the movements of the form with the goal in mind of improving their balance and avoiding the pitfalls of a sedentary lifestyle may represent quite an accomplishment. An additional, perhaps overly demanding, form of Ch'i Kung might push the boundaries of their limits too far. Other teachers may take the approach that the internal aspects of T'ai Chi are to be held in reserve for more advanced students once the form itself has been well learned.

Traditionally, the internal components of many systems were held in secret, until the student had proved his loyalty to the Master or to the style, over untold years of diligent practice. This usually meant no studying with other teachers. This business of withholding information and keeping knowledge secret may sound like the stuff you only see in movies, yet it is wholly congruent with my own experience. Some years back, the T'ai Chi student of another teacher (the teacher having been an older Chinese gentleman) came to augment his studies with me simply as a matter of convenience because of his proximity to my school. Given his previous experience with his other teacher, who taught only the form, this student had lots of questions about Ch'i energy, the manifestations of which he was just beginning to feel as a result of his practice. Reportedly, his teacher when questioned, had denied any knowledge of the internal aspects of T'ai Chi, that is until this student began revealing to him that he was deriving tangible results from the energy cultivation practices he had learned from me. (In China, this student probably would have been dismissed for augmenting his studies with another teacher, but hey, this is America, and times have changed.) At this, the floodgates opened and his teacher was suddenly an authority on Ch'i and Ch'i Kung practices. He had had this knowledge to share all along, but for some reason, probably due to tradition, was reluctant to do so until presented with the prospect of a student who appeared to know more about the subject than he. Again, an approach such as this is quite different from my own approach, but I am reluctant to pass judgment on the teaching styles of other colleagues in my field who, as noted earlier, may have perfectly valid reasons for teaching the way they do. Certainly there are a variety of approaches that can produce good results.

Two Pioneers

The scenario described above, which took place back in the mid 1980's, is increasingly rare due to a change in teaching attitudes, prompted primarily by the wide dissemination of information available today on various Ch'i cultivation and Ch'i Kung practices. I want to take this opportunity to credit two men who each in his own way is largely responsible for this shift in attitudes. The first is Master Mantak Chia who, to the best of my knowledge, was the first to publish comprehensive texts in English on Taoist energy meditation and Ch'i Kung practices. Chia's special gift was his ability to distill esoteric Taoist theory and practice down to a consumer, or lay, level. To date he has produced numerous volumes on various aspects of this work (his earlier works being simpler and more straight forward and direct than some of his later work.) Another pioneer in this field has been Dr. Yang Jwing Ming, a scholar and prolific writer whose work parallels Chia's in many ways. Dr. Yang's work, I am pleased to note, is increasingly ori-

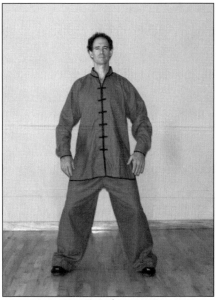

Figure 7-1. Tai Chi Open Stance

ented towards medical Ch'i Kung and is helping to bridge the gap with Western medicine. There are a number of other fine writers out there today, but Master Chia and Dr. Yang were trailblazers, among the very first to present the concepts of Taoist energy work and Ch'i Kung in a way that made sense to the average westerner. Their conviction and initiative, often in the face of criticism from teaching colleagues, led the way, and in fact compelled other teachers to follow suit or risk being left in the dust.

Before concluding this chapter I want to share a Ch'i Kung technique that anyone can practice on his or her own, either as an adjunct to T'ai Chi or as a separate discipline.

SIMPLE STANDING

Probably one of the simplest techniques you can practice offers the combined benefits of several of those areas outlines in previous chapters. Simple Standing is an excellent way to improve balance and to begin to develop a sense of rooting. As a meditation in stillness it can afford relief from stress or tension. And, as a Ch'i Kung practice, Simple Standing will induce the flow of Ch'i through your body's acupuncture channels.

Simple Standing is just that, and it is perfectly safe for all ages. In order to begin practice you can adopt a standard T'ai Chi open stance (see Figure 7-1), adjusting it to be narrower or wider according to your own balance or state of health. As you stand, flex your knees just slightly, torquing them gently out from the center so that the knees are over your feet. Position your arms in front of your chest as if you were creating a basketball hoop, with your fingertips almost touch-

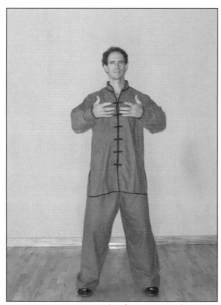

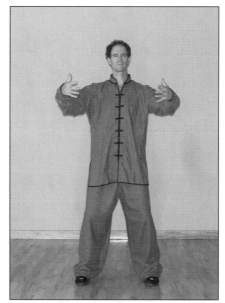

Figure 7-2a. Here the fingers are shown nearly touching...

Figure 7-2b. ...or the fingers/arms may be held wider apart. In either case the chest remains hollow.

ing.[1] (see Figures 7-2 a, b) At the same time, imagine your chest as a sail on a sailboat catching a gentle breeze from the front. This will help you to hollow your chest (concave) and to spread and round the scapulae (convex) in back. Let your elbows *set* as if there were small weights suspended from them. The level at which you hold your arms can also vary according to your skill and conditioning, or even simply according to your preference, as depicted in the photos below (see Figures 7-3 a, b, c).

Now Stand

Start slowly, standing only for brief periods of 3 to 5 minutes at a stretch, depending on your age and ability. For older folks, for whom falling may be a concern, you can stand near a chair back or counter top. Even if you do not need to rely on it, just knowing some support is close at hand can be reassuring. In all likelihood you will find yourself tiring as you stand (probably in the arms and shoulders) long before any of the aforementioned benefits are felt. Gradually over time, you can increase the duration of your practice. The key is to challenge your limits so as to increase them, but not to the point of strain.

You may recall that it is often said of meditation, "the less that happens outside the more will happen inside". This will certainly be the case if you are properly attentive to your own process. If (when) you begin to experience fatigue try not to simply quit. Instead explore that feeling of fatigue. Ask yourself, why do you get tired in one place but not another? What minor adjustments can you make to bring yourself more into proper alignment and thus ease any strain? What is hap-

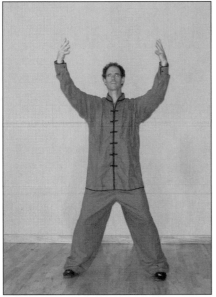

Figure 7-3a. Hands and arms held higher,

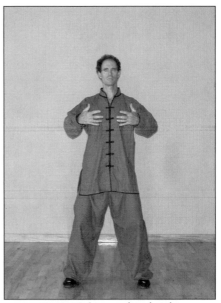

Figure 7-3b. ...at chest height,

pening to your respiratory pattern as you continue to stand? What thoughts, distractions, resistances, or games, does your mind engage in as you stand? Is the discomfort that comes with standing really the same thing as pain? And at what point is it really prudent to surrender to that discomfort?

Gradually over weeks and months of standing you should have ample opportunity to address each of these questions, and no doubt others of your own. You will find that the answers to these questions are variable according to how your practice evolves. By the time you have reached the 10 minute mark you will likely begin to feel some changes in rooting awareness, as well as some feeling of heat (energy) in the body. By 15 or 20

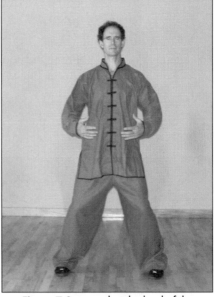

Figure 7-3c. ...and at the level of the Dan Tien.

minutes you will definitely begin to feel more rooted and an awareness of more of a sense of stillness within. I must caution you though not to simply force yourself to stand in order to test my predictions. You must let the process evolve naturally rather than strive to meet some goal or agenda. Such an approach would only prove disappointing. Allow yourself at least several months to build up to the point of standing for periods of 20 to 30 minutes. Be sure to remember that, while it may be true that one benefit of standing is to increase your endurance, endurance is not the goal of this practice. The aforementioned benefits associated with Simple Standing will accrue from practicing until you can relax effortlessly into your standing posture rather than from straining or struggling.

In conclusion, Ch'i Kung in general, and Simple Standing in particular, can be enjoyable and rewarding adjuncts to your T'ai Chi practice both in terms of the benefits they offer directly, as well as in the way they can inspire new insights into your existing body of knowledge.

THINGS TO REMEMBER:

- T'ai Chi is, ideally, a form of Ch'i Kung.
- Ch'i Kung emphasizes mindful and deliberate attention to breathing.
- Ch'i Kung is an ideal way to cultivate your energy to catalyze your T'ai Chi growth process.
- Simple Standing Ch'i Kung is a safe and "easy" practice, enabling you to begin to address the issues of stress, rooting, and Ch'i cultivation.

Notes

1. Depending on personal preference, the distance between your fingertips can range anywhere from 1 to 24 inches. The actual distance between the fingers is secondary to maintaining that feeling of roundness between, chest, arms, and fingers.

CHAPTER 8

Heartfulness and Freedom Through T'ai Chi

"God is a verb, not a noun"
  —Buckminster Fuller

"Know thyself", advised Socrates to his charges.
Asked one student, "Sir, you say 'Know thyself' but do you know yourself?"
"No," responded Socrates, "but I know something about not knowing."

F reedom...
One of the greatest benefits that T'ai Chi has to offer to those who embrace its precepts is the potential to become freer. Freer in our bodies, and freer in our souls, freer of those limitations that would hinder us in attaining our full potential as human beings.

Aspects of T'ai Chi that deal with freedom of the body are amply addressed elsewhere throughout this book. In this chapter I will address freedom of a different sort, that which can be achieved through the development of "heartfulness."

WHERE IS THE HEART IN T'AI CHI?

In other eastern disciplines, the Yogic traditions for example, there are whole branches of practice such as Karma Yoga, Bhakti Yoga, Raja Yoga, and others, all of which deal with matters of the heart and soul in very deliberate ways. These various approaches encompass a range of virtuous qualities such as personal morality, integrity, congruence, altruism, and joy. Surprisingly, there appears to be no corresponding focus of attention as such inherent to T'ai Chi. Any attention given to these virtuous qualities seems merely coincidental to the practice and its reputed spiritual roots. With few exceptions, attention to matters of the heart and spirit is conspicuously absent from the T'ai Chi literature currently available.[1] I find this surprising given T'ai Chi's reputation as a personal development tool.

Please Note: In alluding to matters of the heart, the spirit, and the soul, I am pointedly not referencing to them here as academic or abstract technical qualities such as *Shen* or *Yi*, as they are often thought of in the context of Internal Arts and TCM. Rather, I am thinking of these qualities as being more akin to the self-actualization concept espoused by the renowned psychologist Abraham Maslow, self-actualization as an expression of one's greatest human potential.

In writing this chapter, I wrestled with a number of terms more western sounding than the ascribed Indian terminologies, searching for the one word or term which might suitably encapsulate the essence of these different virtues as they relate to T'ai Chi. I thought of labels such as compassion, insight, charisma, and so on, before finally assigning these qualities to the domain of *heartfulness* because they are potentially dispositions of demeanor (who we choose to be), as much as they are qualities of character (who we are). Since being heartful also encompasses (in my mind) being truly free, these qualities, freedom and heartfulness, seem to me mutually compatible and for the purposes of this topic, synonymous.

STANDARDS OF THE HEART

Perhaps the want of literature addressing heartfulness in the realm of T'ai Chi stems from the very personal nature of the topic. Our paths are unique, and along these paths each of us may or may not choose to confront our own standards of integrity and morality while exploring our potential for becoming fully realized spiritual/human beings. For myself, the issues of morality, integrity, empathy, responsibility, respect and appreciation for life, purposefulness, and joy are inextricably woven into the pursuit of martial arts mastery, and particularly so in the case of internal arts such as T'ai Chi. This is not to say that I consider there to be only one constant standard for any of these qualities, and certainly I do not see myself as the designated arbiter of any such standards.

> I do believe however, that T'ai Chi practitioners have a unique opportunity, and an incentive, to explore and expand their growth. They can develop heartfulness according to their own individual scope by virtue of T'ai Chi's emphasis on integrative mind/body experience through the discipline of practice.

To me, this only seems congruent with T'ai Chi's alleged potential as a tool for mastery of self.

CONGRUENCE AS ONE COMPONENT OF HEARTFULNESS

Personal congruity is the embodiment of wholeness. It is having all your ducks in order, and being on a steady path, even though you may not always be steady on your path. Such congruence, in encompassing many of those qualities identified in the previous section, is one component intrinsic to heartfulness. Heartfulness does not necessarily mean being pure of heart or pure of action, or always knowing what is the right course to be taken. It does mean, among other things, keeping with the desire and the intention to hold oneself accountable for at least a modicum of personal growth along the way. Such congruity is thus a path rather than a destination. Personal congruity, as one more form of process, is a way of keeping to that path.

> This means that if you find yourself involved in a discipline, such as martial arts, which contains an implicit focus on personal development, it would be essentially incongruent, even wasteful, to squander the opportunities for growth afforded by that discipline. After all, what good does it do to practice the T'ai Chi form if, in its fuller manifestation, it cannot inspire peace and joy in a restless spirit in one's daily living?

IMPEDIMENTS TO HEARTFULNESS

Speaking of restless spirits, no discussion of heartfulness would be complete without at least touching on those factors which can typically serve as impediments to being truly heartful. Extenuating circumstances (such as chemical imbalances or congenital mental disorders) aside, Traditional Chinese Medicine recognizes that the *five negative emotions* (grief/sadness of the lungs, fear of the kidneys, anger of the liver, impatience/cruelty of the heart, and worry/neurosis of the spleen), can be prime suspects in tilting the scales of good health against our favor. For someone whose energy is inordinately bound up in any of these emotions the attainment of true heartfulness can seem a distant goal indeed.

I discussed briefly, in Chapter 5, the concept of Displacement, and how too much of any negative emotion can displace its positive counterpart to the detriment of our well-being. If you are someone who is characterologically stuck, (i.e., in anger, etc.) then Tai Chi alone may be of limited value in getting those emotions to release their grip on your inner soul. I do not pretend to suggest that Tai Chi is some kind of panacea; it cannot be all things for all people. Given a clear and deliberate intention/attention on your part, as well as a commitment to the discipline, Tai Chi may, in conjunction with other modalities, be instrumental in helping you to advance measurably along your chosen path. Tai Chi can help you to become 'literally', more grounded to the earth, and by extension, more composed and less frenetic within. Even in cases where individuals may be chronically bound up in their own negative energy, Tai Chi can set ready a stage for heartful progress.

HEARTFULNESS CAN HELP YOUR T'AI CHI

Just as T'ai Chi can set a stage for the myriad qualities of heartfulness in your life, so can the reverse be true. Heartfulness can quite literally improve your practice. In my own training, I cannot help but notice a correlation between my capacity for empathy, resulting from an enhanced ability to both listen and perceive, and my improved level of skill as a push hands player.

In the early 1990's I pursued adjunctive healing studies in Classical Homeopathy. Subsequently, as a lay practitioner of that healing modality I found it necessary to listen non-judgmentally, for one to two hours at a sitting, as clients shared their stories, often baring their souls in the process. My job was to listen for what was said, as well as for what was left unsaid, in an effort to perceive what were the most real and pressing pathologies and wellness issues of the person before me. I emphasize the importance of "perceiving" versus simply listening because what clients really needed to have addressed in their lives often represented a significant departure from what they volunteered in so many words as their chief complaint.

I found, initially, that my background in T'ai Chi helped me to listen and perceive more effectively. I also discovered that as I refined my ability to perceive, and evolved in my own capacity for empathy with my clients, I naturally became more sensitive in other areas of my life, most notably in my physical sensitivity during T'ai Chi Pushing Hands practice. I found myself becoming softer in my touch, more sensitive to the touch of my partners, and more able and willing to listen rather than talk. This happened to a degree beyond that which I would ascribe solely to my T'ai Chi training. My experience serves as an example of how growth of a heartful kind (in my case through my experiences as a health care provider) can have a very direct effect on the quality of one's T'ai Chi practice.

METAPHOR AND TOOL

I do believe strongly that T'ai Chi has quite a lot to offer in the realm of intra-personal growth and personal morality. For starters, T'ai Chi is a metaphor for balance in one's life, and it also represents the epitome of balance in action. In order to be truly balanced, I believe that one must attend to all parts of one's being. The operative phrase here being, *one must attend to*. T'ai Chi is as suitable a tool to accomplish this balance, in all of its facets, as any other self-help modality with which I am familiar.

> In the end, T'ai Chi is just that, a tool like any other, and the finest tool left idle will not produce its own results. Consequently, it is the student's responsibility to ferret out T'ai Chi's subtler gifts and then to use those gifts to their fullest advantage.

It is often the case in our culture that intra-personal growth or self-actualization is synonymous with psycho or spiritual therapy of one sort or another. The reason for this is that growth often results from insights into our deeper unconscious selves. The experience of such insights can liberate us from patterns of thought, belief, or behavior that limit our personal growth potential.

Despite the proven efficacy of therapy with trained professionals many people still prefer to do their own work. However, modalities representing the therapeutic self-help approach are intrinsically limited in their capacity to enable us to perceive credibly below the surface. By definition, that which is subconscious is imperceptible to conscious view and awareness, and as noted in the earlier chapter on Stress, the subconscious quite prefers to maintain its status quo. This is why it is often easier to navigate those depths when guided by a skilled and objective mentor such as a therapist. In the absence of some form of third party intervention, the greater part of who we are usually remains concealed and inaccessible (according to nature's design) in the subconscious realm.

INSIGHT THROUGH T'AI CHI

Nevertheless, we can sometimes under certain conditions or with the right incentive, catch glimpses of what lies below the surface on our own.

> T'ai Chi has the potential to facilitate these conditions and affords us an opportunity to get as closely in touch with our heart of hearts as is likely to happen away from the therapist's couch. T'ai Chi may never replace psychotherapy in this regard, but one of the limitations of talk therapy is that it speaks at best, indirectly to the body. In so doing T'ai Chi can bring to the surface, knowledge hidden deep within the recesses, knowledge that in some cases may be inconveniently more intrinsic to the body than to the mind.

Other non-movement oriented approaches such as meditation can be limited in this capacity as well, and for the same reasons.

Because it involves movement of a nature that is slow and mindful, Tai Chi can enable us to flirt with that boundary between the conscious and subconscious self, so the gap between the two becomes narrower and less opaque. Just as it is widely accepted that there are conscious and subconscious components to the mind, so I believe it is with the body. There are aspects of the body that lend themselves to everyday awareness, but other places where accumulated layers of stress and tension effectively seal off the outside world. Under the right conditions, T'ai Chi can facilitate the possibility for personal insight and inspire direct access to self-knowledge, which is latent more in the physical component of the body/mind.

Despite my embrace of body/mind integration as an overall theme in my own practice and teaching method, the fact is that some people are more of the mind, while others are more of the body. This is in no way incongruent with my premise of body/mind integration on an individual level. On the contrary, the fact that all people tend not to be integrated in the same way is quite natural. It is just another way of saying some people are more yang while others are more yin. It does make for a more interesting world.

Along this line, you may recall my earlier reference in the chapter on Displacement, to our opportunity and very obligation as students of T'ai Chi to become better human beings. "Better" is something of an amorphous concept, as it can have different meaning for different people at different times. "Better" is thus a relative qualifier. Regardless of what comes to mind for you as a manifestation of becoming better, I encourage you to be conscientiously reflective about your own *intention* to become better, in order that you can play an active and deliberate role in your own process. Thus, any change for the better on your part will not be simply inadvertent but will be due to your own initiative, even if yours is just the initiative of thought or belief as opposed to that of action.

GOOD PHYSICAL HEALTH AS A PART OF OVERALL HEALTH

Certainly the idea of being better would seem to somehow tie in with health, with *being* healthy. But there again is another one of those relative qualifiers in the notion of being *healthy*, healthy as opposed to what? How do being better and being healthy relate to this idea of heartfulness and Tai Chi? And what, one may ask, is a better, or even a truly healthy, human being?

I feel that the concept of heartfulness is best realized if as one part of being both physiologically healthy and being of sound mind, that is as an expression of enjoying good health overall in its broadest context. As someone who is committed to being healthy through healthy living, I have long reflected on the question, "What exactly is good health?". The most reasonable and all encompassing definition that I have found as to what constitutes good health overall has been suggested by Dr. George Vithoulkas, founder of the Homeopathic College in Athens, Greece and one of the world's leading Homeopathic physicians. Borrowing Vithoulkas' own definition (with only slight modification) I would describe good health as follows.

WHAT IS GOOD HEALTH?

- Freedom from physical pain stemming from an overall state of wellness and wellbeing.
- Freedom from extreme emotional passion resulting in a dynamic state of serenity and calm.
- Freedom from selfishness, having as a result the ability to contribute creatively to the common good.
- Freedom from spiritual distress and the achievement of resolution as regards universal truth.

Dr. Vithoulkas may be a Greek Homeopath but this definition sounds pretty Taoist to me. I would say that this definition of good health captures the spirit of a very large part of what Tai Chi is all about. It certainly seems to encompass heartfulness as I have been discussing it, heartfulness being one crucial component of overall good health as described above. Heartfulness is not just a state of emotions; it is a state of being, and a goal to be continually striven for, if never attained.

LISTEN INWARDLY TO DEVELOP INSIGHT

As stated earlier, an important quality concomitant to heartfulness is that of insight. Developing your capacity for insight can open many doors in your practice and in your life. T'ai Chi, as well, can inspire insight. Devising exercises to convey experientially the principles of heartfulness within the T'ai Chi context presents its own unique challenges. Scrutinizing your inner self for those places where the opportunity for fundamental change may lie is not quite as simple as examining your root or repositioning your knees. Nevertheless, you can still apply T'ai Chi principles to this task by employing a variant of your *Ting Jing* listening skill (see Displacement chapter). Rather than using your skill to sense an opponent, as would be the case in Pushing Hands or actual self-defense, you will use it here to perceive more deeply into yourself. The internal quietude of T'ai Chi can set a ready stage for this. Just as a cacophony of sounds in the world outside makes it difficult to zero in and focus on any one sound, so can the opposite occur. A state of serene dispassion attained through and during the practice of T'ai Chi can enable you to more aptly perceive the whispering voice of your own inner soul. Some of my most poignant moments in terms of self-realization have occurred while I was deeply engaged in the practice of my T'ai Chi form.

Of course, any discussion of individual personal issues is clearly beyond the scope of this book. However you can begin this exercise logically by asking yourself where you might be somehow unresolved, in conflict within yourself or in conflict with others. Conflict (to be discussed next chapter) is that dynamic which strikes me as most antithetical to T'ai Chi, but "conflict" need not be your issue of choice. You can modify the following exercise, employing its basic format as a model to address any number of issues pertinent to your own growth.

HEARTFULNESS (IN)ACTION

As you begin, first consider that I am not asking you to think superficially about your chosen issue, such as who made you angry yesterday, as part of your exploration around feelings of conflict. I am referring here to deeply held issues around which a lack of resolve somehow creates limitations in your life. Second, you cannot expect meaningful results if you try to implement this exercise in any casual manner, for example while you are reading this book. The idea is to create a context, through your form, in which you can be deeply relaxed and yet remain cognizant of what your body/mind has in store for you. The directions for this exercise are not complicated or overly specific, and there is no right or wrong approach.

In order to sense deeply you have to be deep. Simply put whatever question you may have for yourself "out there" and trust that it will be dealt with once you have relaxed into a more introspective state. You can do this in much the same way someone might seek out answers or guidance for themselves via their dreams. During your form practice, I recommend that you not preoccupy yourself with any desire for insight. Culling insights from the depths of your body/mind is not the same as ordering out for lunch. Your subconscious self will not accede to the demands or agenda of conscious desire except on its own terms, so just put yourself in a good place, and trust the process to unfold as it will during your practice.

As you proceed through the moves of your form, simply be sensitive to any tiny little pains or limitations in your body, whether in the muscles, inside the joints, or in the fascia. Notice any feelings of discomfort or anxiety in your mind. In encountering any such sensations, you can simply be aware of them and move on, or you can linger, sensing for any more meaningful feedback. Sometimes a pain is just a pain, but even small pains can be indicative of more significant issues. Try to avoid analyzing your process as it unfolds and just let it happen. Any time you put something out there you may or may not be blessed with hoped for insights. Insights tend to surface only when you are truly ready for them. Just because you want something, no matter how badly, does not necessarily mean you are ready for it. By removing your ego from the process, in effect letting go, that which percolates to the surface, even if not what you thought you wanted, or if not what you sought, may be the very thing which requires your attention. To borrow a line from the Rolling Stones, "You can't always get what you want. But if you try sometime, you just might find, you get what you need."

Insights around such issues as conflict can reveal themselves in various ways, either as direct awareness, bodily sensations, or as subtle shifts in the way you find yourself in the world. For example, noticing that you have tension in your neck might inspire a recollection of driving in heavy stop-and-go traffic as the apparent cause, which then might remind you of a stressful encounter at work preceding your drive. This in turn, may inspire you to reevaluate your handling of work related stress as the actual cause. You may even find yourself having arrived at some unexpected realization about some more global aspect of your life. Tracing back like this can help you recover useful information from your body that might otherwise remain inaccessible. Conversely, information/insight may not always be as forthcoming as we might like, and that can be its own form of information.

HEARTFULNESS AND INTEGRATION

For those of you who practice T'ai Chi, I think it is fair to say that heartfulness, and the freedom that comes from developing it, are fairly synonymous qualities. If not actually born of your attention to many of the other qualities discussed in earlier chapters, they are concomitant to, and strongly influenced by them. If your practice has included conscientious attention to cultivating your Ch'i, resolution and relinquishment of long or deeply held stresses, and connecting conscientiously to our host planet to develop a root, while attending to the consequences of your actions and behavior according to the principles of displacement, it then follows that you are evolving as regards the qualities of freedom and heartfulness in your own practice. I can think of no better illustration of this than a passage from Stuart Alve Olsen's book, *The Ten Essential Principles of T'ai Chi Chuan*, in which he quotes his teacher, the famous master T.T. Liang as he is just finishing a round of practice. "*Oh, I went to paradise...so happy, I just did the whole form without knowing it...my mind was bright and clean.*"

THINGS TO REMEMBER:

- Heartfulness is a state of demeanor (who we choose to be) as much as a state of character (who we are).
- Heartfulness and T'ai Chi can mirror each other's development.
- T'ai Chi is a metaphor for balance in one's life as well as the epitome of balance in action.
- Insight through T'ai Chi can liberate us from limiting thoughts, beliefs, and behaviors.
- T'ai Chi enables us to flirt with the boundary between our conscious and unconscious selves.
- Insight can happen in our bodies just as it can in our minds.
- As a rule, insights surface only when you're ready for them.

Notes

1. In alluding to matters of the heart, the spirit, and the soul, I am pointedly not referencing them here as academic or abstract technical qualities, i.e. Shen or Yi, as they are often thought of in the context of Internal Arts and TCM. I am thinking of these qualities as being more akin to the self-actualization concept espoused by the renowned psychologist Abraham Maslow; self-actualization as an expression of one's greatest human potential.

CHAPTER 9

Conflict—An Antithesis to T'ai Chi

"The blue mountain is the father of the white cloud.
The white cloud is the son of the blue mountain.
All day long they depend on each other,
without being dependent on each other.
The white cloud is always the white cloud.
The blue mountain is always the blue mountain."
　　　—Dogen

If someone were to engage me in one of those word association games—"Say the first thing that comes to your mind when I say...T'ai Chi"—my likely response might run the gamut from "slow", or "peaceful", to "quiet", or "fluid", or "balanced", or some such thing. The one word least likely to come to mind would be "conflict". To me conflict represents a state of being which is wholly antithetical to T'ai Chi Ch'uan. However, the discussion of conflict is apropos to T'ai Chi to the extent that conflict is self-realized and can limit the fuller development of our body/mind potential as T'ai Chi enthusiasts, but only if we allow it to do so.

WHAT CONFLICT IS, UNIVERSALLY SPEAKING

In truth, conflict is just a human concept for a human condition. There is no corollary for this elsewhere in the universe (or so I presume). In reality (another human concept) there is just Tao. The Tao is not real, it is just the Tao.

We humans tend to perceive conflict as an absence of harmony, as being out of balance with the Tao. On a grand scale the universe knows no such conflict: there is Tao. What we might ordinarily regard in our universe as conflict, (Stellar bodies exploding, meteors colliding, what have you) can more accurately be described as "opposing", rather than conflicting forces. Opposing forces in the universe always beget harmony, because sooner or later they always manage to resolve to a state of balance, the only variable being one of scale. Such forces are an inevitable part of the ebb and flow of the 10,000 things. In the grand scheme of things, the interaction of opposing forces would seem to be a part of universal homeostasis, and is a means by which the Tao maintains harmony and relative stability within its realm. Thus the only "real" conflict in the universe exists in the hearts and souls (and bodies) of men, and then only because we make it so.

OPPOSITE OR CONFLICTING

Opposite or opposing forces are not the same as conflicting forces, which promulgate disharmony, i.e., conflict between two persons. Opposite forces exist in abundance throughout the universe. Our universe is made up of and held together by these very forces. Opposite forces always exist in a state of relative balance, and it is their mutuality which serves as the most basic premise of Taoism and of T'ai Chi. Yin and Yang, front and back, above and below, hot and cold, all are examples of opposites which, not only exist in harmony, but in fact owe their existence to their relative opposite.

Opposites both attract and serve to complement each other, as can be seen in the case of opposite magnetic poles. Try this—take two magnets and attempt to connect the positive and negative (opposite) poles. The magnets will attract each other and get along just fine. But if you try to force the two positive poles or the two negative poles together, the result is conflict, not because their forces oppose each other, or naturally repulse each other, but because you are trying to force something that is not natural. Thus, conflict happens when two opposing forces encroach upon one another in a way that fails to respect their natural flow. One of the goals of T'ai Chi is to learn how to transform conflicting forces to opposite and balancing forces, thus restoring harmony.

FREE WILL

The relationship between opposite forces that I have just described manifests most obviously on a cosmic scale, often for unfathomable cosmic reasons. We can also see examples of both opposite and conflicting forces at work in the human realm. With regard to the manifestation of these forces in the human realm, there is one other important variable to be taken into account, that of free will. Of all the forces in the universe, humans alone can be said with any certainty, to have the capacity for free will. For human beings then, free will is usually the operative factor in determining whether any two forces are merely opposite or conflicting. Just as our free will can open many doors for us, so can it be used to close doors. Much of the conflict we experience in our daily lives stems from limitations and stricture, as well as from an inability or unwillingness to listen so as to recognize when we are displacing or being displaced. This keeps us from being rooted to our earth and to ourselves, which in turn imbalances our Ch'i, and so on, and so on. Thus the inertia of conflict can perpetuate itself unless we exercise our free will to take some initiative in recognizing and adjusting the daily patterns of our lives. In the end, nobody can make us feel conflict except ourselves.

Conflict is an internal dynamic that is generated in response to an intolerance for some real or imagined internal or external stimuli. One can create conflict within one's own body simply by attempting in the wrong way to relax and stretch muscles held taut due to chronic tension. For example, you may want your waist to turn one way and perhaps your back refuses to cooperate, opting instead to strain a muscle or subluxate[1] a vertebra, resulting in pain. Pain, in this case as the manifestation of conflict between two opposing forces, might possibly have been avoided by listening more closely in order to perceive the body's limits, and by adjusting your practice goals accordingly.

How Conflict Affects Us

Conflict affects us adversely to the extent that it limits the ability of our bodies and our minds to operate freely. The body/mind, you may recall from the earlier chapter on Stress, always acts in what it believes to be its own best interests. In this sense, we are agenda driven to protect our interests. First and foremost on our agenda is survival. After survival, most people's agendas include food, clothing, and shelter, all our basic needs. These alone have proved fodder for conflict on a massive scale throughout the ages. Humans always seem to have been vested in the belief that conflict can be employed effectively as a means of restoring (their own) harmony even when at the expense of the harmony and well-being of others. Most obviously, such conflicts have manifested in the form of war and violent crime. For humans, as sentient beings with a capacity for free will, conflict can also manifest on a smaller, more personal scale. In responding to any presenting conflict, internal or external, the body/mind's first and most normal (learned) response is to protect itself by retrenching. This again is the sympathetic nervous system's fight or flight response at work. The body predictably responds to conflict by tensing up. The mind has its own preferred defense mechanisms, creating blockages or walls, ostensibly to insulate itself from any perceived danger. For the mind the response can take the form of neurosis, maladjustment, aggression, etc. Ironically, in seeking to protect itself from external conflicts the body/mind often succeeds in perpetuating its dilemma with compensatory acute or chronic internal (intra-personal) conflict, which may be perceived by the body/mind as the lesser and more manageable of two evils.

Conflict Pandemic

When I stand back and look at the state our world is in today, I am disturbed by the pervasive reporting, pandering actually, of conflict in the various media. As a consumer I am also saddened by the attention accorded the media, stemming from peoples need for direct or vicarious experience of conflict as a form of narcotic reprieve from the pain and unwanted challenge of their own truly deep and unresolved personal crisis and turmoil. More simply put, misery, even subtle misery, enjoys company. This may sound melodramatic, but I do not believe that I am overstating the point. More often than not, people are totally unaware of their own deeper issues.

A popular example of this dynamic comes to mind in the role played by actor Matt Damon in the movie *Good Will Hunting*. I opt to invoke his character, Will

Hunting, as an exemplar of inner conflict. Damon's character portrayed a regular guy, an otherwise bright and well-adjusted young man, who was always on the edge of acting out violently in response to his own unresolved inner demons. I thought Damon's character was both easy to relate to and believable. The sort of intra-personal conflict he displayed is much more common than most people might imagine. Such conflict can variably manifest as acts of emotional or physical violence inflicted on others, or it can fester as an internal dynamic never quite surfacing but exacting its toll on one's physical, mental, and emotional health.

NOT BEING "OUT" OF HARMONY

The esoteric purpose of T'ai Chi is to bring ourselves more into harmony with the Tao. Being "in harmony with the Tao," really means not being out of harmony with the environment, the world in which we live or with those we encounter. Most especially, it means not being out of harmony with ourselves. Often, people think being in harmony with the Tao is some *state of being* which is beyond their reach and which must be arduously pursued. This calls to mind for me the term "health food", misnomer that it is. Food is by definition already healthful, at least until we start processing it or adding other stuff to it. In the same way, people are by definition part of the Tao, only losing the feeling of connectedness once their lives become "over processed" with too many additives. Of course, not being out of harmony also implies our being able to restore harmony if we temporarily step from its path, as inevitably will be the case from time to time. Temporary missteps aside, we cannot simultaneously be in a state of harmony and be stuck chronically, in even a low-grade state of sympathetic excitation. Thus, one of the higher goals of T'ai Chi practice is to learn to neutralize and balance those forces, internal or external, that would conflict us.

STEP BACK FROM CONFORMITY

All too often people feel helpless to implement the changes necessary to free themselves from self-imposed conflict. This propensity to feel out of control is often rooted in social mores, which is not surprising given the cultural impetus for conformity. One powerful example of this is the way we are brought up to believe in the sanctity of science as the arbiter of nature's laws. We are taught that what goes up must come down, carcinogens cause cancer, sugar causes tooth decay, fire burns, and so on. These are the facts of life. When we accept these precepts as law, without question, it precludes our exercising free will to participate in life more fully as an open-ended affair.

The universe is an ongoing creative process. With our free will, we humans can choose to participate in that process or not. Though it is not specifically related to T'ai Chi, I will nevertheless tear a page from my own book in sharing an experience that proved profoundly enlightening for me as regards the transformation of intra-personal conflict. I can think of no example that more graphically illustrates the power of free will in the arbitration of conflict than the ritual of firewalking. This is because each of us "knows" that fire burns. We know it in our minds, and most of us have also had some confirming experience in our bodies that fire does indeed burn: the lit cigarette, the hot stove, the spilled coffee, etc. For most people the experience, along with the belief that fire burns, has been seared into our body/mind in more ways than one. Thus it would seem to be an exercise in conflict to deliberately embark on an experience that we know causes pain and suffering.

FIREWALKING AS A METAPHOR FOR CONFLICT RESOLUTION

Back in the mid 1980's, I was invited by friends to participate in a firewalk, which turned out to be the first of many. If you are not familiar with firewalking, it involves a brief period of body/mind preparation which leads up to walking barefoot across a bed of hot coals heated somewhere in the range of 1300 degrees Fahrenheit. Despite repeated efforts of the scientific community to debunk this ancient ritual, I can attest that there is no trick involved. Skeptics have offered a host of logical reasons to explain away this phenomenon, such as, "insulating ashes afford poor conductivity of heat," and so on. But I have witnessed individuals stroll out to the middle of a bed of red hot coals, to stop there and stand while scooping up handfuls of flaming embers for what seemed minutes on end, then calmly step from the fire with even the hairs on their feet unscathed by its heat. The scientific validity, or absence thereof, of firewalking aside, there is no denying that standing barefoot at the edge of a bed of hot coals is a potentially provocative experience. Assuredly, this activity is not without a great deal of risk as I have also been witness to others burning seriously. Given the risk involved, and the fact that firewalking is not likely to be rated highly as an asset on one's resumé, one question begged is, "Why do it?"

As one might expect, the experience of actually walking across hot coals barefoot without burning is quite profound. It serves as unmistakable evidence that we can indeed move beyond the boundaries of nature assigned us by science. If one can exercise enough initiative to "bend" the laws of nature (to change our beliefs, in effect), even if just for a few brief moments, what then are the other possibilities? What other (self-imposed) limitations present in our lives might we be able to move beyond? Of course, the other question that surfaces is, "How is it that ones does not burn?"

My friend, Michael Sky, author of *Dancing With the Fire,*[2] believes that a burn is nothing more than a manifestation of conflict. If one were to come inadvertently into contact with fire, in contrast to one's intention to do so (two conflicting forces), the result would be a burn. "Getting burned" is in fact a euphemism often used to describe the aftermath of many different kinds of conflict, including those of the internal kind which leave us feeling "burned out". However when someone steps deliberately onto a red hot bed of coals with a clear "attention" and an equally clear "intention" to not burn, somehow the basis for conflict can be neutralized. Attention/Intention is an extraordinarily powerful force. The purpose of firewalking is to teach us that we can exercise our free will in expanding beyond those limitations normally ascribed us, and that foremost among those limits is conflict. T'ai Chi can serve as a similarly effective (albeit less sensational, though somewhat more practical) means of moving beyond the limitations of conflict, external or internal.

CULMINATION IN SUMMARY

What I have written so far in this chapter on conflict is again, a culmination of the information provided in my earlier chapters. Whether you are reconciling the issues of stress and tension, exploring the challenges of finding your root, mediating the forces behind displacement and envelopment, or exploring for heartfulness and insight, the successful negotiation or avoidance of conflict is crucial to your mastery of T'ai Chi and mastery of yourself. Only you, with your capacity for free will, can take the initiative in assuming responsibility to this end. In a very profound way, "learning" T'ai Chi is at best, an applied study in conflict resolution/avoidance. Whereas "knowing" T'ai Chi, means simply having evolved to a place where mind and body are, by normal standards, free of conflict's limitations.

THINGS TO REMEMBER:

- Interaction of opposing forces is part of universal homeostasis.
- The mutuality of opposite forces serves as a basic premise of Taoism and of T'ai Chi.
- A goal of T'ai Chi is to balance opposite forces to restore harmony.
- Free will can determine whether two forces are opposite or conflicting.
- Conflict is an internal dynamic generated by intolerance for real or imagined stimuli.
- Attention/intention is extraordinarily powerful in neutralizing/transforming conflict.
- Learning T'ai Chi is, among other things, an exercise in conflict management.

Notes

1. To misalign or dislocate, as a vertebra.

2. Michael Sky. *Dancing with Fire.* 1989

PART 2

INTERMEDIATE/ADVANCED THEORY AND TECHNICAL PRACTICE SKILLS

CHAPTER 10

Miscellaneous Practice Hints from the Ground Up and from the Outside In

Notwithstanding my earlier seeming indictment of the western orientation towards mechanics and reductionism, I will use this chapter as an opportunity to share some of my own T'ai Chi insights from a more detailed technical perspective. The mechanistic/reductionist model is not inherently bad, it only becomes a problem for T'ai Chi players when it excludes other potentially valid perspectives. In the case of T'ai Chi, narrowing your scope to better understand the mechanics of body positioning and placement can actually be quite helpful in grasping many of the finer points.

One of the idiosyncrasies of assessing relative competency in many fields of study is that new students are often credited according to what they have learned and how they have improved their skill. In contrast, more advanced students and teachers tend to be assessed inversely, according to whatever desirable qualities remain conspicuously absent from their knowledge or practice. So it is with T'ai Chi. "So and so is a very good teacher, if only he could get his root." "Too bad Master so and so has bad knees, sticks out his butt, holds her chin too far forward," etc. In this chapter we will cover a number of miscellaneous points. Some points will indirectly facilitate improved technical performance, such as in the section on Tai Chi stretching. We will also address more directly, many of those small but critical areas that often get touched on during the course of instruction, but not necessarily in a sufficiently concise or comprehensive manner to produce significant or lasting improvement. By attending to these areas of your practice you can hopefully avoid having said of you, "(S)He is very good, but...!"

STRETCHING FOR T'AI CHI

It is my experience that the emphasis placed on stretching and flexibility practices in T'ai Chi varies widely from teacher to teacher. I believe that stretching and flexibility practices are vitally important for opening up the body. As I alluded in the earlier chapter on Stress, stretching can work for you or against you, depending

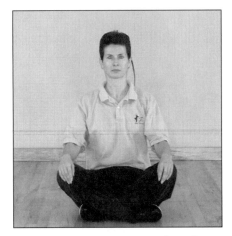

Figure 10-1a. Sitting cross legged and upright.

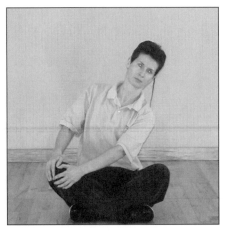

Figure 10-1b. Begin by opening the body to one side, slowly, vertebra by vertebra and rib by rib.

on the approach you take and on the way that approach affects any baggage stress you may be carrying. There are many credible approaches to stretching, and the one(s) you choose will depend on exactly what you are attempting to achieve. If you are stretching with the idea in mind of relinquishing stress and tension from the body and of opening up the body and expanding its limits, then I recommend a slow mindful approach, versus something more rigorous. A slow and mindful approach to stretching will be quite compatible with your own T'ai Chi practice. It represents an approach to stretching which I view as being not so much some-

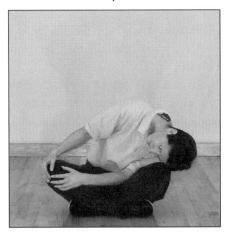

Figure 10-1c. Surrender to your breath, letting your body succumb fully to the effects of gravity.

thing you *do* as it is something you simply facilitate and *allow* to happen. Ideally this can become one more example of doing by not doing.

To get started, you will want to create a context for yourself that requires minimal initiative on your part, one in which you can allow the process to take over so that you can trust gravity to exert its influence on your behalf. You can use this following stretch to open your ankles, knees, hips and waist, intercostals, shoulders, and neck, first on one side of the body, then on the other. Begin by sitting cross-legged, and clasping either knee with both your hands for support (see Figure 10-1a). Let your body gently lean off to the side opposite from the knee you are clasping (see Figure 10-1b). Once you have reached the limit of your lean, pay close attention to notice where it is that you are feeling limited. Use your mind to direct your breath into that place of limitation. Feel the breath gently and gradually filling and displacing any tightness. Then as you allow the breath to be released, *allow* your body to open up a little farther (see Figure 10-1c). Stay with this position, *allowing* your body to melt beyond its limits, for as long as you feel comfortable, anywhere from several breaths up to fifteen or twenty inhalation/exhalation cycles. Breathe into tension, then release and relinquish as you exhale. You can do the same with any place in your body that feels tight or uncomfortable.

In deference to students or populations such as the elderly or infirm, for whom stretching on the floor might be inconvenient or impractical, the same stretch can be modified in such a way that it can be practiced while sitting upright in a chair, preferably one with arms for safety. The breathing remains the same as do many of the benefits. You can practice this modification as follows.

Sit on a chair with your feet flat on the floor and your back straight (see Figure 10-2a). Being careful to avoid as best you can any leaning forward or backward from your back or waist. Begin by sinking your right elbow down toward the inside of your right waist. Simultaneously feel your left shoulder and elbow rise up (see Figure 10-2b). Continue sinking the right elbow, now more to the inside of the right groin/thigh area. As you do this begin to raise the left elbow (left arm bent) up over the left shoulder. Feel the two elbows stretching away from each other as if you were pulling your arms apart. With practice you will become proficient to the point that you can align the left elbow plumb over the right elbow as if there were a string passing straight from the left elbow through the left fist, through the right fist, and on down to the right elbow (see Figure 10-2c). As with the aforementioned floor stretch this exercise will compress one side of your body (right) while expanding and opening the rib, intercostal, and shoulder area on the other (left) side. Recover to a sitting position, relax with a few breaths, and then repeat to the opposite side.

These approaches to stretching are akin to peeling an onion, slowly stripping away thin layer after thin layer of underlying tension, gradually moving deeper and deeper. The idea is to avoid even thinking of stretching in the usual goal oriented way, but rather to think in terms of allowing the body to regain its natural freedom of openness by simply letting go of anything that prevents or interferes with its being more flexible. Throughout this process your breath will be your best ally. As you recover from any such stretch, be sure to stay connected with your breath so as to minimize reliance on the very muscles you have just relaxed. In sending a message to your muscles and soft tissues that it is safe to release and open up beyond previously held limits, it is important that you not then undermine the rapport established with those tissues by calling them immediately back into play lest your muscles tense up and defeat the very purpose of slow and mindful stretching. Once you have completed one side of a bilateral stretch, take a

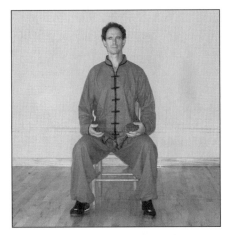

Figure 10-2a. Sitting upright

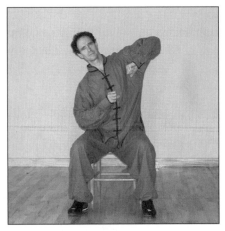

Figure 10-2b. Leaning to one side to sink the elbow while raising the opposite shoulder.

few quiet breaths while sitting upright or standing. Use this opportunity to sense for any changes or discrepancies in how you are holding your body before proceeding to stretch the other side. With this approach as a model, you can apply this method of breathing, releasing, and opening to almost any other stretch you practice.

WHAT IF IT HURTS? STRESS DISCLAIMER

In the earlier chapter on Stress, I discussed in some detail the psychosomatic challenges of relinquishing stress from the body/mind. I would like to add one other cautionary piece of advice in

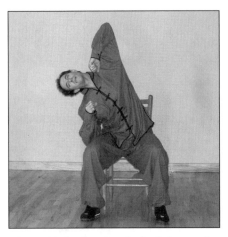

Figure 10-2c. Opening the body by stretching the elbows apart.

preparing you for possible after effects of this work. As you begin to strip away the body's more superficial layers of stress and tension, you may find that underlying layers of tension, now exposed and unprotected, will leave you feeling physically sore and achy, mentally spacey, or emotionally vulnerable. As your body progressively relinquishes its layers of protective armor, you may even find yourself revisiting or recalling those long forgotten issues that caused your stress to accumulate in the first place. In case of discomfort of this kind, versus pain from injury, it may be necessary to rest your body for a day or two. Remember as you do, to keep breathing into your discomfort. Any pain or discomfort which fails to self-resolve within a couple of days may require the attention of someone skilled in dealing with soft tissue trauma, such as a chiropractor or massage therapist. Gradually, as your body acclimates to the challenges of expanding beyond its old limits, the likelihood of discomfort following stretching will diminish as well.

I always ask new students, when enrolling at my school, to disclose any pre-existing musculoskeletal issues or health care concerns. Back problems are by far the most common musculoskeletal problem for people today. It is usually the case that students with pre-existing problems feel initially worse for a few classes as their body's superficial armor is peeled away leaving the underlying and more sensitive areas exposed and vulnerable. In most cases two to four weeks of participation in T'ai Chi is sufficient to realize significant improvement and freedom of movement over previous limitations.

Stay Within Your Limits

As long as I am on the subject of disclaimers, it bears mentioning that the expectations and standards you hold for yourself should be appropriate to your age and to your state of health. Younger and healthier students at T'ai Chi will have physiologies that allow for greater demands on their physio-adaptive capabilities. Older students should not be dissuaded in their efforts toward T'ai Chi mastery but should remain particularly mindful of working *with* their bodies, rather than against them. Over time T'ai Chi really can change your body at a level deeper than that of the superficial musculature. Some of the changes T'ai Chi conduces will occur at the level of your tendons, ligaments, and even your bones. You will find that even these deeper components can be strengthened and made to be more resilient as a result of your practice. Connective and skeletal tissues can indeed develop in accordance with the demands placed on them, but remember, the phrase "over time" is operative here. Bones, tendons and ligaments are essentially avascular and as such, they tend to heal very slowly when pushed too far or too fast. So for best results, keep your stretching practice slow and steady and regular.

What to Do with Your Toes and Feet

Your feet are where you connect to the earth; an obvious but oft ignored bit of trivia. In T'ai Chi, your feet will establish a foundation for everything above. Thus if your feet are mis-aligned, no amount of upper body compensation can make things right. There are a number of different stance positions in T'ai Chi, but the most common is the forward leaning stance (a.k.a. Bow and Arrow stance), or variations thereof. Again, actual stance and foot positions may vary slightly according to teacher or style, but as a rule it is important to not cross the lines of your feet when in this stance. That is to say, if you were to straightedge an imaginary line through your front foot, from its middle toe back through the heel, the imaginary line extending backward should pass well to the inside of the heel of the back foot (see Figures 10-3a, b, c, d). A common error of many beginners is to flare the front toes outward so that the same drawn line would intersect

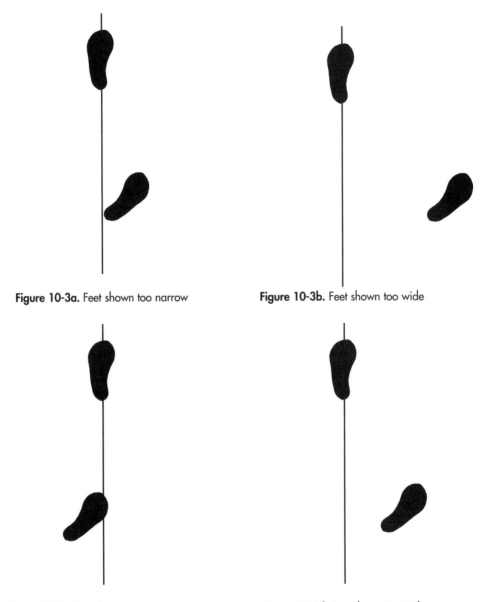

Figure 10-3a. Feet shown too narrow

Figure 10-3b. Feet shown too wide

Figure 10-3c. Feet shown way too narrow

Figure 10-3d. Feet shown just right

the back foot (bad), or worse, pass to the outside rather than the inside of the back foot. In such a case your stance would be overly narrow. An error such as this in standing, will render your Qua susceptible to collapse and undermine your stability overall.

The back foot in this stance should be angled with the toes turned outward anywhere from thirty to forty-five degrees, (see Figure 10-4) the exact angle to be

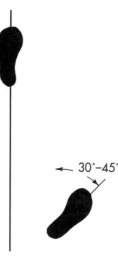

Figure 10-4. In most cases a 30–45 degree angle is appropriate for the back foot.

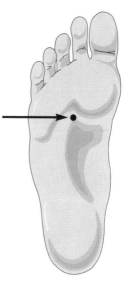

Figure 10-5. Bubbling Well Point, aka Yung Chuan, aka K-1.

determined by how the waist and upper body are oriented. During your T'ai Chi practice try to keep both feet down flat to the earth except for those obvious positions in which the toe or the heel is raised or the leg lifted by design.

In addition to familiarizing yourself with the Bubbling Well point, (see Figure 10-5) pay attention during practice to the quality of your connection to the earth via your nine contact points (see Figure 10-6). These points are the five toes, the outer blade edge of the foot, the heel, the ball of the foot, and the small ball located behind the fourth toe. These are the points that would leave footprint marks were you to walk across rice paper or hard sand. As these are your contact points to the earth,

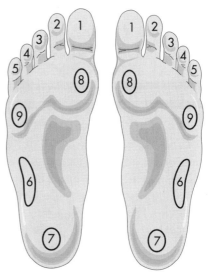

Figure 10-6. The Nine Contact Points.

you must rely on these points in order to issue self-generated force efficiently outward, or when transferring the incoming force of another person either downward to the earth or safely past your own body.

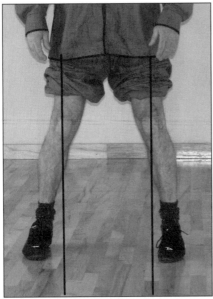

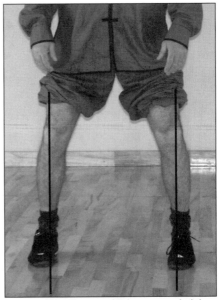

Figure 10-7a. In this photo the knees are not aligned over the feet as they should be.

Figure 10-7b. Here the knees are slightly torqued out so as to be properly positioned over the feet below.

What to Do with Your Knees

As a general rule, you will want to keep your knees slightly flexed and aligned over your feet. The key word here is "slightly", as over bending the knees will engage the quadriceps muscles to the point that the legs become reliant on muscular force rather than structural connection. Assuming you are standing up straight in an "open stance" with the feet parallel, flex your knees forward to just over the toes, and feel them turned ever-so-slightly outward so as to create a gentle torque on the inner thigh (see Figures 10-7a, b). This opens the Qua (see Figure 10-8a). Conversely, turning the knees inward would pinch the Qua shut, and reduce the opportunity for pelvic articulation. In order to feel how this works, you can experiment with an exaggerated pelvic tilt as follows (see Figure 10-8b). Stand as described above, and rock your pelvis front to back, noticing how freely you are able to move. Then, turn the knees inward and try rocking in the same fashion. Compare your range of motion. You will note that the range of motion is clearly more constricted with the knees turned inward. If on the other hand, you were to make the mistake of turning your knees too far outward, beyond the point where the thighs align parallel over the feet, your insteps and heels would tend to peel up and pull the body forward and off balance.

In deference to women, I must add that there is credible evidence that the physiology of the female pelvis, being typically wider than that of males, may require some modification of the advice given in the previous paragraph. According to W. Norman Scott, M.D., Chief, Division of Orthopedics at Beth

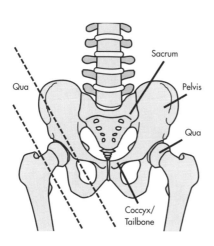

Figure 10-8a. The Qua, regarded generally as the loin/groin area, refers specifically to the inguinal crease.

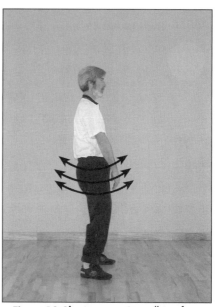

Figure 10-8b. An open Qua allows for a greater range of motion when rocking the pelvis.

Israel Hospital, N.Y. in his book, *Scott's Knee Book*, the alignment of the female femur, as well as the tibia below it, may dictate separate consideration. A female T'ai Chi teaching colleague of mine shared the following account,

> *For over five years I've lived with uncomfortable knees. The pain was becoming worse and my mobility was increasingly impaired until I considered surgery. I decided to discover why T'ai Chi was aggravating instead of healing my condition. I began to move slower in my practice, paying closer attention to where, when, and how pain occurred as I moved. What I learned was that my knees like to be "in" slightly and that this allows more freedom in my hips and in my lower back. After just a couple of months of changing the way I position my knees during practice, they are free of discomfort. If I revert to my old "slightly outward" position of the knees, the pain returns.*

The above account notwithstanding, I stand by my earlier recommendations (as for most of my female students this is a non-issue), but encourage women who do feel discomfort in their knees to feel free to experiment with their positioning, preferably in collaboration with their teacher or medical provider.

THE PERINEUM (*HUI YIN*)

[Please refer to the Glossary for an anatomical description of the Perineum and its significance to internal practices.] It is quite important to keep the perineum

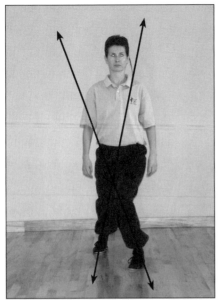

Figure 10-9a. These three photos depict the principles of knee alignment as they apply in the Leaning Stance. This photo depicts an overly narrow Forward Leaning stance as evidenced by the crossed lines.

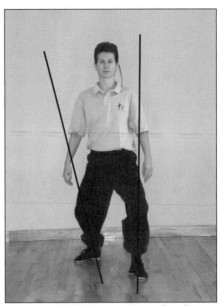

Figure 10-9b. By comparison this photo depicts a Forward Leaning stance which is too wide due to the flaring of the back knee and the front foot.

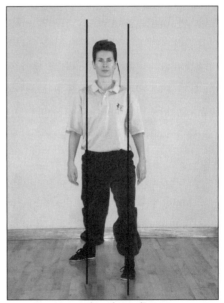

Figure 10-9c. This photo shows a correct position with the feet, hips, and shoulders all properly aligned.

(*Hui Yin*) aligned directly below the crown point of the head (*Bai Hui*) in order to maintain good T'ai Chi posture. To accomplish this you will need to develop a more conscious and ongoing awareness of the perineum (see Figure 10-10). Otherwise, alignment of the perineum will probably become one of those qualities that you believe to be theoretically important, but only because you have been told it is so. One way to really get to know your perineum is to find an old tennis ball (or a rolled up sock), position it under your perineum, and sit on it. (The old Masters used biscuits.) Practice this "sitting meditation" whenever the discreet opportunity presents itself, and you will find, almost immediately, that your posture becomes more properly aligned and your awareness of your perineum more automatic. I always keep a couple tennis balls on hand, even in the car, for just this reason (caution: when driving do not lose your tennis ball under the pedals—not funny).

During your practice of the T'ai Chi form you will want to relax the perineum to the point that it feels to be the floor for all the internal viscera above.

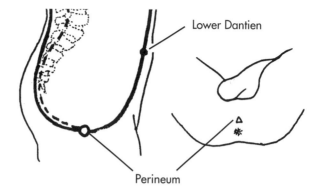

Figure 10-10. The Perineum includes that area forward of the anus and back from the genitals.

WHAT TO DO WITH YOUR QUA

You will recall from earlier discussion that the term Qua refers to the inguinal crease just inside each hip (see Figure 10-11). An inflexible Qua is the bane of any T'ai Chi student, as it precludes the waist's firmly connecting together the upper and lower halves of the body.

If you stand with your hands placed over the ball joints of your hips and alternately rotate your knees inward and outward, you will observe that there is a clear connection between the movement of your knees

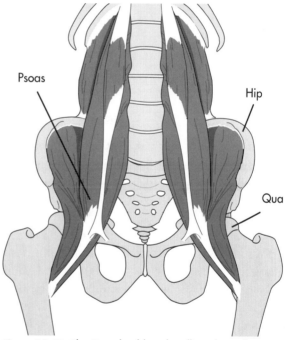

Figure 10-11. The Qua should not be allowed to collapse in Tai Chi.

and that of your hips. Now reposition your hands over the Qua just inside each hip, and repeat the same motion. Once you are familiar enough with this articulation, to distinguish automatically between a closed versus an open Qua, you can pause at random points in your form practice to check that the Qua is, in fact, being held open. For those readers whose orientation is more martial, I assure you that maintaining an open Qua is not tantamount to leaving the groin area exposed and vulnerable.

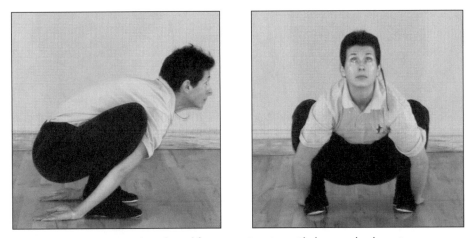

Figures 10-12a, b. Side and front view. Pressing with the arms back against the shins to open the Qua.

An exercise which I have found very helpful in developing that quality of an open Qua is to squat down low with both feet flat. Position your feet about shoulder width apart and flare your toes slightly outwards. Now open your knees as wide as possible, (see Figure 10-12a, b) and let each of your arms reach from the inside of the thigh down and out to the side around the ankles. Continue reaching with both hands, extending them back along the outside of each foot. Be sure to keep your palms facing upward as you press the backs of your hands down against the floor, so that the insides of your upper arms push firmly back against your shins. To optimize this stretch, raise your chin upwards as far as possible, reaching for the heavens with your gaze. You can hold this stretch for as long as you are comfortable. If you do this correctly you will feel the press of your arms against the inner thighs prying open the Qua.

A somewhat more challenging version of this stretch is to sit on the floor with your feet flat down and drawn in together. Pull your knees up toward your chest and then let them flop outwards to the side. Then with your arms positioned inside of your knees, reach your hands far enough forward so that you can extend your elbows under your shins. Pull back with your elbows against your shins (as if you were trying to crawl forward through your own legs) (see Figures 10-13a, b). The idea is to get your feet pulled back near enough to, or even under, the perineum so that you can shift your body forward from a sitting position up into a squat while keeping your feet flat. This is all done without needing to use your hands to push off the floor (see Figures 10-13c, d). Good luck with this one. This stretch is very good for opening and connecting the entire /waist/lower back area.

THE ROLE OF THE WAIST

The waist can be regarded as that wide belt-like section of the body that extends from the level of the naval downward to the level of the hipbones. Thus it

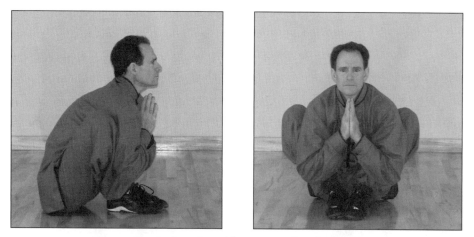

Figures 10-13a, b. Side and front view with tailbone on floor.

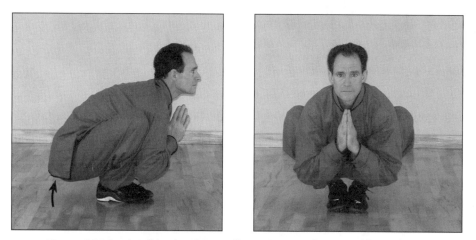

Figures 10-13c, d. Pull back with your elbows into your shins to rise from a sitting position into a squat position. (No hands.)

actually includes the aforementioned Qua. In T'ai Chi, the waist is regarded as your steering wheel. The waist determines what direction the upper body faces and serves to connect the lower body with the upper body as a single, albeit segmented, unit. Consequently, the role of the waist is closely tied to that of the Qua below and the tailbone behind. All upper body power and force must transfer through the waist. In this sense, the waist functions as the mechanical equivalent of an electrical transformer station in that it can receive and store power from the lower body (briefly) before releasing it out to the upper body for maximum efficiency. This process can also be thought of as roughly analogous to the manner in which nerve impulses accumulate their electrical charges prior to crossing a synapse. Only once a sufficient charge has built up during the resting potential can a threshold be reached, at which point the nerve impulses cross over the

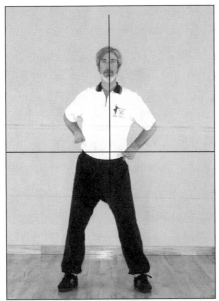

Figure 10-14a. One hip higher than the other. Notice how this upsets the nose-over-navel alignment.

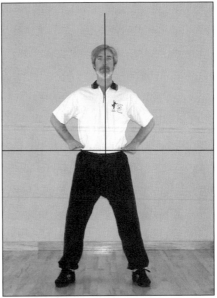

Figure 10-14b. Here the hips are correctly level.

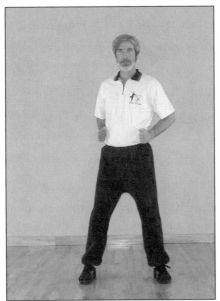

Figure 10-15a. The direction of the finger/palms reveals the hips to be twisted out of alignment.

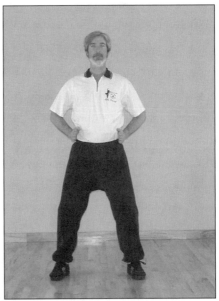

Figure 10-15b. Here the hips are properly straight.

synapse fully charged to continue on along their path. Thus the power and force generated by the muscles and structure of the lower body move in a similar manner through the waist to be released out through the upper parts of the body.

Two common errors often made by new students, or by those suffering from low back pain or spinal imbalances, are to inadvertently tilt the waist up or down to one side or to the other, or to twist the waist out of its alignment with the upper or lower body. In some people these tendencies can be quite marked. In the first case (one side higher than the other) this can be revealed by placing one's hands, palms down, against the upper ridges of the pelvis (ilium) and by comparing their relative height while standing before a mirror (see Figures 10-14a, b). In the case of side to side misalignment, (again using a mirror) the hands can be placed with the palms flat against the hips and the fingers pointed straight ahead (see Figures 10-15a, b). Make any necessary adjustments in order that the hips, waist, and upper and lower body all match up in the direction they face. Serious or chronic misalignments may require the attention of a chiropractor or bodyworker.

WHAT TO DO WITH YOUR TAILBONE

As noted earlier, the tailbone can articulate forward and under or back and out, provided the Qua is sufficiently open to allow for this to happen. I have worked with teachers whose approach emphasized an exaggerated positioning of the tailbone, alternately curled well under or tilted way back. If you are a beginner it may actually be helpful to experiment with this exaggerated approach, (see Figures 10-16a, b) but only until you gain some skill at positioning the tailbone on demand. When sinking the weight back from the forward leg into the rear leg in any stance, imagine that someone has attached a pull line to your tailbone so that the tailbone leads the way in drawing the whole of your body backward while the spine is kept plumb (see Figure 10-17). Conversely, curl the tailbone slightly under as you move forward. Feel your tailbone as if it were providing the very impetus for forward motion, driving the body before it. I often liken the tailbone/sacrum, to use an automotive analogy, to "rear wheel drive." Once you have acquired a reasonable command of this tailbone skill, you will want to understate, rather than exaggerate its application in any positioning of the tailbone. Too much curl or tilt will actually weaken your tailbone connection.

THE KIDNEYS

As mentioned in the earlier chapter on Ch'i, the kidneys have bearing on T'ai Chi in respect to their role of storing of *Jing* and of governing the bones. In addition, they are located in close proximity both to the waist and to the center of the body. According to TCM theory, the kidneys tend to run cold, overly so in the case of deficient *Jing*. Consequently, you should *sink your Ch'i* into the lower abdomen and thus fill the kidneys with warm energy by breathing into them, not to the point that the surrounding muscles tense up, but to the point that you feel the kidneys are full and connecting down to the tailbone.

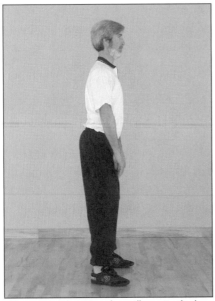

Figure 10-16a. Here the tailbone is tilted to the back, exaggerating the lumbar lordosis.

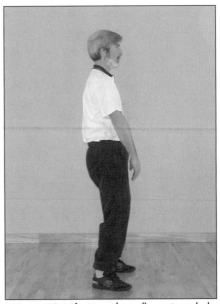

Figure 10-16b. Here the tailbone is curled too far under, causing the shoulders to slump forward.

WHAT TO DO WITH YOUR SPINE

The spinal column is an amazing structure. It houses the Central Nervous System in all its delicacy, yet it can facilitate the transfer of incredible power surges in to or out from the body. The spine is like a drive train extending upward from the waist/tailbone. It can be used whip-like to deliver snapping force, or it can be held somewhat more rigidly to facilitate the delivery of whole body shocking power, or it can twist and turn to evade attack or deflect an incoming force. Despite its inherent flexibility, the spine can be vulnerable to injury even under benign circumstances. T'ai Chi can help you develop more resilience in your spine and its surrounding soft tissues, thus decreasing the likelihood of

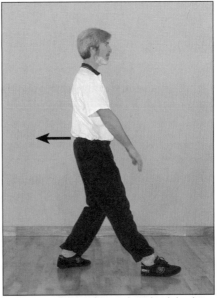

Figure 10-17. When sinking back let the tailbone draw the body as if it were being pulled by a string.

inadvertent injury. As a general rule, the spine should be maintained fully elongated and erect and ought to be regarded as somewhat analogous to the central axis of a revolving door around which the rest of the body moves (see Figure 10-18).

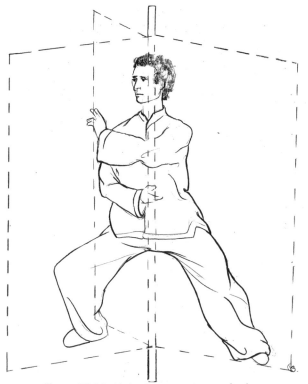

Figure 10-18. Maintain your spine as plumb.

WHAT TO DO WITH YOUR BACK AND CHEST

Your back and chest are two sides of the same coin. The Classics advise "sinking the chest, raising the back," etc. This is often misconstrued and interpreted too literally. The problem for many people is that chronic upper body stress in the trapezius muscles, causes the shoulders to hunch up and round forward. In some cases, tension in the back will draw the scapulae, commonly referred to as the shoulder blades, together creating tightness in the upper back (see Figures 10-19a, b). In order to position this area correctly for T'ai Chi, begin by opening the axillary (underarm) area as if you were holding an imaginary tennis ball under each armpit. Ease the shoulders downwards as you do so. (Any tightness in the trapezius muscles will make itself felt here.) Meanwhile, imagine your chest as a sail on a sailboat catching a gentle breeze from the front. This will help you sink the chest (Slightly concave), (see Figure 10-20a) and simultaneously separate the scapulae in back (Slightly convex) (see Figure 10-20b). This separation is necessary in order to engage the scapulae against the rib cage. This is a must if you are to facilitate any efficient transfer of force between the arms and the rest of the body. You might find it helpful to think of the scapulae as "front wheel drive" in comparison to the tailbone/sacrum's rear wheel drive. (Note: I personally prefer four wheel drive.)

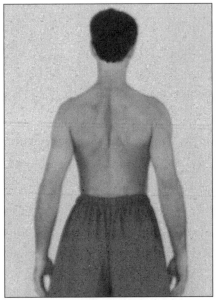

Figure 10-19a. Tightness in the back causes the scapulae to be pulled back and pinched...

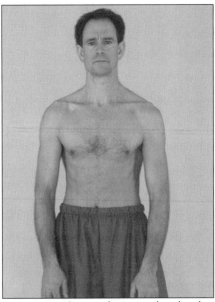

Figure 10-19b. ...And armpits closed to the point that the arm-to-scapulae connection is weakened.

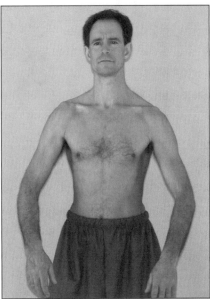

Figure 10-20a. Here the chest sinks and the armpits open...

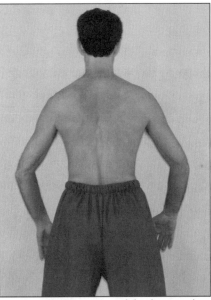

Figure 10-20b. ....Meanwhile, the scapulae separate, allowing the back to round some-what, establishing a structural link between the arms and the rest of the body.

WHAT TO DO WITH YOUR ARMS AND HANDS

The role of the arms in T'ai Chi can be underscored by imagining in your mind's eye how your form would feel or appear if you lacked arms at all. Somehow your T'ai Chi would just not be the same. The arms are critical for balancing the body as well as for issuing outgoing power and negotiating any incoming force from an opponent.

Of course the wide range of arm movements and postures occurring in the form precludes specific instructions here for exact positioning. However the arms ought to be kept relaxed and free of tension (See chapter on Stress—Divesting Yourself of Stress and Tension Held in the Body). When the arms are extended outwards, the elbows should be kept slightly bent as if there were a small weight suspended from each of them (see Figure 10-21). This will help to insure the integrity of both the arms-to-scapulae connection and the elbows-to-tailbone connection. As a general rule, the arms will each be governed in their movement by their connection down through to the opposite foot. Force traveling through the right arm will emanate from the earth connection at the left foot and vice versa.

If you were to liken the progress of any wave-like force that is traveling through the body to be released out through the arms, to that of the snap-

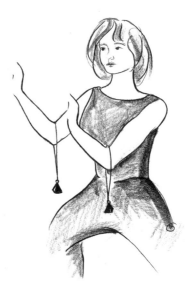

Figure 10-21. Here the arms are extended with the elbows "set" as if there were a small weight suspended from them.

ping force of a wet towel, the arms and hands may be thought of as the towel's striking tip. The impact of such a strike would be rendered less devastating if the last few inches of the towel were heavily starched to the point that the wave of force was disrupted rather than smooth. Any tension in your arms will similarly undermine the smooth transfer of force. For this very reason the arms must be kept relaxed, but not limp, in order to facilitate the efficient release of power. Using the example of a towel, it is easy to visualize how a force would travel (if you imagine the towel unraveling in slow motion), wave-like, through to the tip. With the human body, unlike a towel, there are rigid skeletal components to be taken into account. Consequently, the action of force traveling through the body is actually more one of unfolding than one of unraveling. Nevertheless, by keeping the body and arms free of stress and tension, this wave-like effect can, for all intents and purposes, still be achieved as the body unfolds naturally with the force

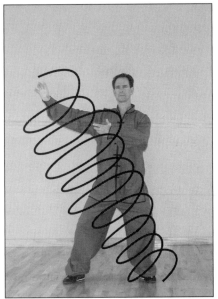

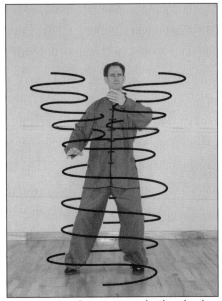

Figures 10-22a, b, c. Feel force spiraling from the earth up and out through the body as depicted in the Wave Hands Like Clouds move.

Figure 10-22b. Wave Hands Like Clouds (continued).

of release (see Figures 10-22 a, b, c).

The wrist, palms, and fingers should be maintained as soft yet sensitive and alert. Pay particular attention to the *Lao Kung* point at the center of each palm (see Figure 10-23). In attending to this point, you can imagine breathing through it and you may actually feel it pulsing. If and when you feel a sensation of breathing or pulsing at the palm, it may be accompanied by another feeling of the fingers themselves as if they were extending distally to become longer, depending on how you execute certain moves (see Figure 10-24). As the fingers extend out you may notice this extending feeling traveling back through the wrist as well as all the way up the arms. Given that there are no muscles in the fingers, this feeling

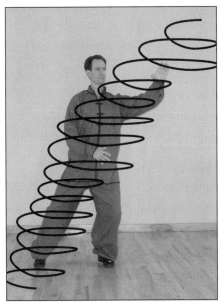

Figure 10-22c. Wave Hands Like Clouds (continued).

of extension will be due to the flexion of the tendons in opening the phalangeal joints. This may be accompanied, as well, by feelings of Ch'i manifesting as heat/energy/tingling at your palms. Visual inspection may reveal a mottling effect on your palms and fingers.

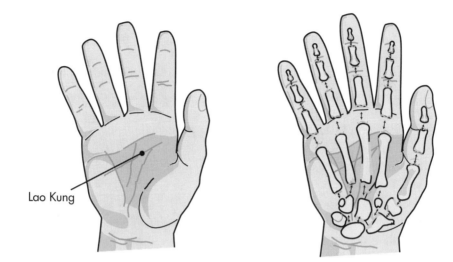

Figure 10-23. Lao Kung Point.

Figure 10-24. Open the palm and feel your fingers extend from the inside out.

HOW TO REALLY RELAX AND SINK THE SHOULDERS

Relaxing one's shoulders, is, unquestionably one of the most challenging tasks for many students of Tai Chi. In today's world so many people carry that world squarely on their shoulders, and it shows. In my experience as a teacher, there is no place where chronically held stresses and tension are more readily and widely apparent in students than in their shoulders. This is a matter of great concern given that the arms cannot function optimally in complying with Tai Chi principles if the shoulders are unable to cooperate.

This dynamic can be difficult to address since the shoulders do not usually "just store" tension. The stress held in one's shoulders is generally more reflective, than is stress held elsewhere in the body, of who someone is, as well as the lifestyle they are invested in leading. For example, shoulders which are held tautly back and down could hint at an aggressive or impatient nature or at a lifestyle in which one is always rushing to get places. Conversely, shoulders positioned chronically forward may suggest that someone is guarded or depressed or perhaps that their lifestyle entails much hunching over books or desks. These various aspects of oneself, as expressed through tension in the shoulders, may be called into question above and beyond the issue of shoulder tension per se.

Your shoulders serve as both a seat for and as a means of protecting, your vital head area which houses your cognitive and emotional functions as well as your primary sense organs. Shoulder tension may accumulate in the first place as the body's best (albeit misguided) effort to stabilize and protect this vital area in response to personality traits or lifestyle issues such as those cited above.

Therefore, letting go of tension from your shoulders can challenge more than just your ability to relax certain muscles. (see chapter on Stress).

Like the waist, the shoulders serve as something of a transfer station coordinating action and information between the head, body and arms. Sinking and relaxing the shoulders is, therefore, crucial in connecting the upper body, through the lower body, down to the earth.

One of the easiest ways for me to communicate to you how to get that feeling of truly sinking your shoulders, is to invoke your memory of a fairly common experience, that of trying to retrieve an object dropped just beyond your reach, perhaps underneath a sofa or table. You know, when you are too lazy to get off your chair and get down

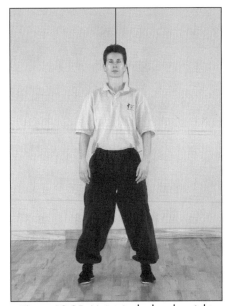

Figure 10-25. Maintain the head upright with the Ba Hui crown point aligned directly over the Hui Yin perineum point.

on your hands and knees to look for it. If this has never happened to you before, then now may just be the time for you to toss your car keys or a favorite earring (or if you are really serious about this, the TV remote) under whatever furniture is at hand. Make sure whatever you drop is just beyond your grasp. Then reach for it. Pay careful attention as you do so, to the manner in which you (would otherwise unconsciously) distend your shoulder downwards for those extra few inches of ("Almost got it") finger stretch. In experimenting with this you may initially feel as if you are straining your shoulders more than relaxing them. If so don't worry. The idea is to really explore your limits for your shoulder's "sink down" feeling. Afterwards, when practicing your form, be sure to relax, rather than strain, to sink the shoulders down. Not only will this exercise serve as a model for how to sink your shoulders down during form practice, it will also teach you how you can sink your shoulders as a means of getting below someone else's root (which is a good place to be if that someone else happens to be an opponent).

WHAT TO DO WITH YOUR HEAD

Your head like your spine, can move according to four planes, forward or backward, turning to the left or right, tilting down from side to side, or elongating upward or contracting downward in the fashion of a turtle stretching or retracting its neck. Generally, the head should be held erect during T'ai Chi practice, as if it were suspended by a string from above (see Figure 10-25). It should sit

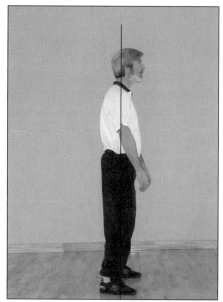 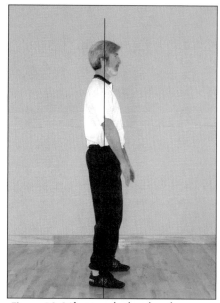

Figure 10-26a. Here the head is held too far forward. Notice the ears positioned forward of the centerline.

Figure 10-26b. Here the head and ears are properly centered in alignment with the perineum and feet.

squarely over the shoulders so that the *Bai Hui* point at the crown aligns directly over the *Hui Yin* point at the perineum.

With tight shoulder and upper back muscles so common today, many people tend to hold their heads overly forward (see Figures 10-26a, b). Of course, imbalances such as this simply serve to bolster any tightness in the shoulders and upper back as these muscles become chronically engaged to stabilize the head as best they can. This kind of imbalance can be self-perpetuating and debilitating. The further forward of center the head sits, the more the supporting muscles need to engage in order to compensate for the downward pull of gravity. As these muscles continue to develop in response to the unhealthy demands placed on them they become ever less able, and willing, to support the head in a proper vertical alignment.

Because most of our sense organs and many of our proprioceptors are located in the head, this is an exceedingly difficult pattern for one to overcome on one's own. Our head serves as a "headquarters" for taking in the information that determines how we perceive our world. Therefore, we can be quite invested in leaving our head right where it is, thank you very much.

In my own case, I came to finally get this particular lesson in a rather unorthodox way. Earlier in my T'ai Chi career, before I had any real sense as to how to recognize tension, let alone relinquish it from my body, I was at a point where I was already holding a good bit of chronic stress in my neck and shoulders. As a result, my head was always too far forward, leading the way. Try as I might, and despite the advice of my teachers, I just could not seem to get a sense of

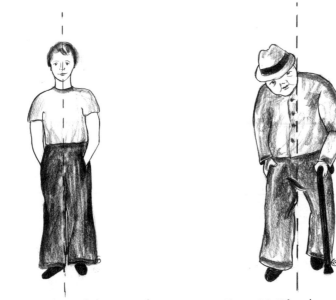

Figure 10-27a. Tai Chi can help prevent this from...

Figure 10-27b. ...becoming this

maintaining my head upright. Then one day, as I was rushing mindlessly to complete a task immediately prior to teaching class, I incurred a painful neck strain, which compelled me to hold my head perfectly still and upright. Not being one to miss a teaching session, I proceeded to teach my class. I realized in the process of teaching that for the very first time I was holding my head correctly and moving it as an extension of my body and waist rather than as an independent appendage. From that point forward I was able to remain more conscientious about the positioning of my head.

For many people, a lifetime of stress can be too much to overcome. I can recall when I was just a teenager, my father stood straight at six feet tall. But, he neglected to take good care of his body. The result was that before he passed away at the relatively young age of sixty-five, he had literally shrunk by some three inches. This is not an uncommon occurrence for people, as they grow older, after a lifetime of accumulated stress and tension. Stresses and tension, left unchecked, can wreak havoc over the long term (see Figures 10-27a, b). The effects of chronic stress and tension in the neck and back in particular, can be insidious. As noted earlier, I am a proponent of modalities such as deep tissue massage or chiropractic intervention as a means of relinquishing stress and alleviating its symptoms. These various modalities can be useful adjuncts to anyone learning T'ai Chi.

Before moving on to the next section, I want to note one other helpful point for you to pay attention to—your nose. During T'ai Chi practice, the nose should be kept in line directly over the navel to insure that any side-to-side turning of the head stems from the waist rather than from the neck. In this manner, if the waist turns, the nose turns, and if the waist does not turn, neither does the nose (see Figure 10-28).

WHAT TO DO WITH YOUR TONGUE

As regards the tongue, there are two considerations to be taken into account. The less esoteric of the two has to do with the role of the tongue in stimulating salivary secretions in order to prevent the mouth from becoming dry during practice. Very simply, this is accomplished by keeping the tongue touching against the upper palate. The tongue also plays a key role, energetically, in linking the body's two major acupuncture meridians, the Conception Vessel (*Ren Mai*) and the Governing Vessel (*Du Mai*). This link allows the Ch'i to flow

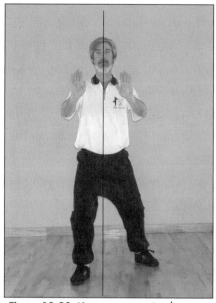

Figure 10-28. Keep your nose in alignment over the navel.

through the body in a complete circuit (Microcosmic Orbit). For the purposes of T'ai Chi, it is of little consequence where exactly on your palate you choose to place your tongue, as long as the contact feels comfortable. Keeping your tongue pressed lightly against the roof of your mouth during practice may seem a bit contrived at first, but with a little practice this will come to feel quite natural.

WHAT TO DO WITH YOUR EYES

For most people, your eyes are the primary means of accessing and conveying information to the brain for neural processing. The eyes are hard wired directly into the body's autonomic nervous system, the role of which is to determine whether our most appropriate response to any given stimuli stems from the sympathetic (fight or flight) or parasympathetic (relaxation response) branch of the Central Nervous System (CNS). The eyes can also convey emotions, spirit, and intention. These combined qualities manifest as *Yi*, which can serve to guide your Ch'i. The eyes can also perceive what they are looking at either directly or peripherally, as when you see something out of the corner of your eye. Of additional import is the role the eyes play in helping us maintain our sense of balance (to check this out for yourself, see how long you are able to stand balanced on one leg with your eyes closed).

When practicing T'ai Chi, it is best to keep your eyes soft but alert, as if you were wearing an expression of gentle kindness. Eyes that are squinting or glaring are not soft. The eyes actually play quite a substantial role in determining the degree to which the surrounding facial muscles become engaged. You can try experimenting

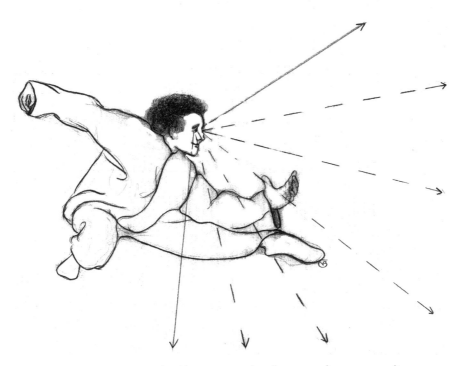

Figure 10-29. Your eyes should remain peripherally aware of your surroundings.

with different "looks" or expressions, in order to feel for yourself how the eyes influence the involvement of facial muscles. Eyes that are clear and soft will minimize tension in the local muscles, which in turn signals the rest of the body to stand down and relax. Given the role of your eyes as a venue for expressing *Yi*, combined with your desire to maintain a rooted connection to the earth, it follows that the eyes also play a role in rooting. Beginners often make the mistake of watching (versus following) the movements of their hands with their eyes to the point that their "looking" undermines their root. Certainly the eyes can follow the hands, but they should retain at least a peripheral awareness of the earth (see Figure 10-29). In T'ai Chi we always employ the least (optimally efficient) amount of effort necessary for any given action. This goes for the eyes as well.

HOW TO BREATHE IN T'AI CHI

My students often ask me, "What is the best way to breathe?" This question always calls to mind an experience I had as a beginning T'ai Chi student back in the 1970's. I had asked my Sifu at the time the same question. He responded, "Breathe naturally." "Thank you," I said, realizing in that moment that I had no idea whatsoever, what he meant by his words. He was Chinese, with a limited command of English, and to this day I do not know if he really meant what I thought it was he might have meant to say. Did he mean by "breathe naturally", to just not concern myself with the breath? Did he mean to breathe abdominally, or was "breathe naturally" a sort of 'code word' meant to imply some special form of respiration? I never did find out. Nowadays, when one of my students asks me what is the correct way to breathe, I always relish the opportunity to wax inscrutably in my reply, "Breathe naturally." Of course, I go on to explain in detail about the implications of various approaches to breathing, but the fact remains that the question often begs more of an answer then the asker expects.

Ideally, breathing should be just as my first Sifu described it, natural. Babies and toddlers do not need to be told how to breathe. They breathe naturally, using their entire bodies to do so. For young children, breathing is natural and spontaneous. It is only as we grow older and feel the weight of the world upon our shoulders that we forget how to breathe naturally, opting instead for more constrained breathing patterns.

The T'ai Chi form actually affords us an ideal venue for natural breathing, providing the body/mind is capable of breathing in a non-compensatory fashion, that is to say, in a manner not dictated by stress or tension. When the moves of the form are practiced correctly, the lungs are exercised like a bellows. Yang (expansive/forward) movements have out-breaths, and yin (contractile/sinking) movements have in-breaths. It will not be necessary for you to already have good breathing skills prior to undertaking any study of T'ai Chi. If you have unhealthy or constrained breathing, that is all the more reason to get started. With continued practice, T'ai Chi can assist you in learning how to breathe more fully. You will find that your breathing can also be employed in a deliberate fashion to help open your body in those places where it is stuck or limited. While practicing your T'ai Chi you can breathe into tightness, into joints, into discomfort, etc, to open your body for a greater freedom of movement.

Once you have begun to relinquish residual tension from the body/mind, you will find that the movements of the form automatically regulate your breath in an optimally efficient manner. Soon your body will breathe you for you, and you will find that it's easy to just "breathe naturally."

Before exiting the topic of breathing I must add that there can be more to breathing than *just breathing* as we usually regard it, at least when it comes to T'ai Chi. What I mean to say is that for most people breathing simply entails the inhalation and exhalation of air into and out from the lungs. But T'ai Chi breathing is that and more. T'ai Chi practitioners should expand their concept of breathing to include the respiration of Life Force energy via the *Yung Chuan* (Bubbling Well) points at the soles of the feet and the *Lao Kung* points at the palms. You can even feel as if you are absorbing energy into your body through the pores of your skin, so that your body really is breathing you. Of course, this level of practice is generally beyond the scope of beginner level T'ai Chi. Even as a beginner though, it is never too soon to start to think in terms of what is possible. Just as a great tree starts from a small seed, so do most of the skills you develop in life start with some form of conceptualization.

In Conclusion

T'ai Chi can be likened to a puzzle comprised of several hundred pieces. If any one piece is missing, regardless of the piece, the puzzle remains incomplete. In that sense each of the pieces has equal billing. Certain "key" pieces do stand out in clueing you in to how to connect apparently disparate parts to make the puzzle whole. The areas that have been covered above represent similarly important pieces, your grasp of which can lead you to develop practical insights about the remaining pieces in your own T'ai Chi puzzle.

Despite the sequential presentation of the practice pointers above, it is quite important to understand that T'ai Chi mastery is not a linear process. It is not simply a matter of getting all the pieces in the right places. Each time you go back to review and reexamine your old learnings there exists a potential for new technical insights and further improvement. Just as importantly, T'ai Chi can inspire an enhanced capacity for insights of a personal nature that can then take seed and manifest within your T'ai Chi form practice.

CHAPTER 11

Optimize Your Practice

In this chapter I have included what I hope will be some helpful training tips in order for you to optimize your understanding of material you may have already learned. The information in this chapter has been drawn from my own personal experience over the years and is shared here based on my dual perspective as student and teacher.

How We Learn New Skills

Over the last thirty-five years I have had occasion to work with many fine teachers, often in intensive workshop settings. It is on such occasions that priceless little bits of knowledge can often be gleaned and stored away for future reference. I know that in my case, it was one thing for me to absorb such knowledge cognitively. It became another thing entirely, for me to actually integrate that knowledge in order for it to become a predictably replicable part of my own practice. Some rare students are gifted in their ability to perceive new information cognitively and then to recall it in their bodies almost immediately on demand. For most of us, such information must be ingrained via repetition in order to become thoroughly automatic and an indelible part of who we are. There is no substitute for the innumerable hours of practice, which can sometimes verge on drudgery, when it comes to actually "getting it", and actually translating the information you have absorbed cognitively into an enduring and replicable body/mind experience.

Repetition Is the Key

Think back to when you were first learning to tie your own shoelaces, a learning process that at that time likely required extraordinary concentration. Years later, you learned to drive a car, always with two hands on the wheel. Not long after that, you probably learned how to sign and balance a checkbook, no doubt with extreme caution at first. Now you can carry on a conversation while lacing those designer athletic shoes, drive while you read the paper (not recommended), and sign checks like they are going out of style without ever looking down. In each case, the task referenced required a great deal of practice to get it just right, but once the skill became ingrained thoroughly, it was there for you whenever you needed it. Repetition breeds familiarity and is the way by which the body commits new learnings to long-term storage (Sometimes referred to as "muscle memory") for recall and instant access. Familiarity in turn, makes things seem easy.

Putting in those hours and hours of practice is the only way for those learnings to become truly yours, until eventually, you earn title to them.

If the world were a perfect place we could read about some desired skill and "presto" we would have it. More realistically, you need to start somewhere when learning a new skill for the very first time. If you are a beginner, cut yourself some slack by remaining cognizant of the fact that the only thing that lies between you and real expertise is practice, lots and lots of (correct) practice.

New learnings are typically absorbed in their most basic and least detailed form. As you continue to review and practice your new learnings over and over and over you will begin, eventually, to embed them into your body/mind to the point that they do indeed begin to become automatic. This then will enable you to focus increasingly at a deeper and more detailed level. In striving for T'ai Chi proficiency, it will become necessary for you to develop a sophisticated command of minutia, such as articulating and opening joints, and arranging and mobilizing disparate body parts with precision and synchronicity. Only once you have developed a thorough command of T'ai Chi in its grosser form, will this be possible. Yet, it is this ability to attend to fine and exacting details, which you can eventually accomplish through diligent practice, that distinguishes the more advanced practitioners from those who are less skilled.

Feel Good, or Feel Right

Everybody has his or her own way of practicing, but for most T'ai Chi students practice means working on the form. For most of the practitioners I know, students as well as teachers, a practice session typically entails a short bit of warming up, followed by a round of form work, with maybe some sitting or standing meditation added in for good measure. There is nothing wrong with this approach. It is an approach I often opt for in my own practice, and it leaves me feeling great afterwards. However, there is the rub. Feeling great and actually making substantial progress in terms of improving your skill level, can be two different issues entirely. If you always feel great, then you probably have failed to address any problem areas latent in your form (assuming of course, that you have not already reached Master level). It is very easy to play to your strengths and to do what leaves you feeling good, but that is not always the same thing as becoming more skilled at what you do. It may actually be a good indicator when you feel as if you have taken a step backwards in your practice, when you feel you have come up against some problem that begs your attention. It takes discipline to shift your attention from your strengths in order to focus on your weaknesses. Therein lies an opportunity for real improvement, if you take full advantage of it.

Balancing Your Strengths and Weaknesses

When you practice the entire form, there will naturally be movements or sequences within the form at which you are more skilled, or movements that you just seem to enjoy more. These moves may beg disproportionate attention during practice. The tendency can be to indulge your strengths at the expense of addressing your weaknesses, causing your strengths to become stronger and your weaknesses, by relative comparison, weaker. It is easy to get stuck in a mode like this and wallow there unaware, never advancing to the pinnacle of your true potential. There are a number of ways you can avoid falling into this training rut. Two of the best ways I know to get more improvement out of your own practice are to challenge your understanding of the knowledge you already have by experimenting with it in altered contexts, and to take into account your optimal learning style. I have included directions below on several different approaches to enhance your training perspective for overall improvement. The training variants that follow immediately will be most appropriate for intermediate to advanced level practitioners. In addition, the section on learning styles will be of interest to anybody, regardless of level.

APPLYING THIS TO YOUR FORM—DIVIDE AND CONQUER

One simple way to avoid getting stuck with permanent strengths AND weaknesses is to divide the form into smaller more manageable sections so you do not lose the trees for the forest. Sometimes when we have learned things, even at a more advanced level, we fall into the habit of practicing them in only one particular way. By so doing, we deny ourselves the opportunity for a fresh perspective. This may be acceptable for a beginning student, for whom everything is already still fresh, but if you have been at your practice for some time, remember that T'ai Chi is not supposed to become one more rigid pattern in your life. It is designed to open up opportunities for becoming freer of limiting patterns, and for living your life in reflection of that freedom. Here is how to proceed:

Instead of practicing the form in its entirety, choose just a move or two on which to work. Practice just that one small piece repeatedly, being careful to not take any aspect of that move for granted. Take it apart, dissect it, and analyze it, as if you were encountering that move critically for the very first time. Hold your position still and notice which muscles, tendons, and bones are involved while you try to feel and maintain your internal connection and alignment. Explore for that exact place, that interface, where the intention of your mind (which is immaterial, and by extension, insubstantial) manifests as a material (and by comparison, substantial) action, executed by your body. Keep in mind as you do this, that interface is an ongoing dynamic process, versus a static event. Once you are satisfied that you have learned something of value and relevance to your training, proceed to the next move and repeat the process. Before going on to a third move, go back and practice the first two moves together in sequence. Examine them afresh now in relationship to each other. Do the same with a third move before tying it back to the previous two. This training approach can be quite time consuming, so a few moves at a time will be ample for any given practice session. This method will generate new insights into old material, thus adding to your depth of knowledge.

ALTER THE CONTEXT

Another approach is to alter the context of individual moves. Many of the moves, as they appear in the form, are practiced only on one side. Any T'ai Chi move can lend itself to bilateral interpretation; whatever move you do on the right side you can also do on the left side and vice versa. Try taking an individual move, or a small sequence, and devise a simple transition, which will allow you to perform the move or sequence first in one direction, and then to repeat the same movement or pattern according to its mirror image, all the while staying in place. Continue back and forth and so on.

Once you have gotten both sides down comfortably you can challenge yourself further by changing the context incrementally. Begin by expanding the move, enlarging it beyond the limits of its usual range, reaching and opening in an exaggerated manner to test and challenge your limits. Pay attention to the way this affects your root, your body structure, your breathing, and the openness and resilience of your soft tissues and of your joints. Gradually, recover back to a normal expression of the movement. From there you can slowly transition to a complete reversal in scale of the just-practiced exaggerated pattern. Adjust the same move to become progressively smaller and closer. Minimize the external motion necessary in order to maintain this move's identity, while you continue to maintain a sense of internal connectedness.

Within either of these contexts, you can experiment further by going slower than normal, faster than normal, or lower than normal. Pay attention throughout, to your root, your balance, your structure, etc. Scrutinize your body for a more detailed understanding of what your limits are and where they lie. By both exaggerating and consolidating, as detailed above, you will develop new and valuable insights into the very same T'ai Chi movements that you have been practicing all along.

CREATING DRILLS

Just as any move from the T'ai Chi form can be interpreted according to its mirror image, so can individual moves be excerpted from the form and sequenced into drill patterns. The less expert your command of any given move, the more you stand to benefit from this training exercise. In the previous exercise you practiced your moves bilaterally in a stationary format. Now you will again alternate from your right to your left sides with the same move, over and over, but this time as you advance along a forward path. You can vary your pace, advancing very slowly (good for those T'ai Chi leg muscles), or you can accelerate to fighting speed, all the while continuing to monitor your internal attention to postural alignment, transfer of force, etc. Pay particular attention that you not bounce up or lunge forward beyond your ability to maintain a root. When moving forward, stay rooted to the back foot. When retreating, stay rooted to the front foot. In this manner, you will become more versatile in your ability to adapt. Eventually you will be able to retreat or practice moving to any direction without compromising your usual practice skills. The greater your command of knowledge about something, and the better you actually know it in your body, the more flexible you will become in your ability to adapt that which you have learned in response to new demands or changing circumstances.

REVERSE PRACTICE

If you are a T'ai Chi teacher, you may find reverse practice (as distinct from mirror imaging) to be very helpful in addressing the training needs of your advanced beginner to intermediate level students. Students at this level often have a fairly competent recall of most of the moves comprising the form. Usually such students will feel most competent with the earlier sections of their form. Those moves are the ones that they have practiced for the longest time and with the greatest frequency. Often students at these levels will have "gray areas" around transitions, or around more difficult or advanced moves. It is perfectly reasonable for those moves that are easier or older to be more thoroughly ingrained in the memory. By always practicing from the beginning, students will reinforce whatever practice pattern they have grown accustomed to, again reinforcing both their strengths and their weaknesses.

In reverse practice, rather than starting your form from the beginning move, and proceeding in the usual sequential manner, you will choose a starting point closer to the final move of the form, or closer to the end of any chosen section in the form, and then perform the last two or three moves only. Just one round of these moves will suffice. From there readjust your starting point back another two or three moves from where you just began and again proceed forward to the end move. Then back up another few moves, and so on. In this manner, by the time you have completed a round of practice, you will have performed the moves at the beginning of the form only once or twice and those moves further along into the form increasingly more. Because this can be such a time consuming process, you may want to experiment with just individual sections at a time rather than the form in its entirety.

This practice method actually represents the reverse of that manner in which most students learned their form, a few moves at a time from beginning to end. By practicing like this, you will actually alter the manner in which the form sequence has been hard wired into your brain. Once again this will discourage any tendency for your T'ai Chi to become just another rigid pattern. Like most other problems or endeavors which we encounter, altering the context can inspire a fresh (in this case, less linear) perspective, and consequently a better understanding of your practice overall.

MIRROR IMAGING

One other fairly obvious approach to mastering your form is to practice it, in its entirety, according to its mirror image. I have known some teachers for whom this was a no-brainer, and I have met others for whom this approach was surprisingly novel. I am a firm believer in bilateral practice when it comes to exercising the mind or the body. Of course practicing the form according to its mirror image will be of greatest benefit for those students who already have a solid command of basic, one sided practice. There is a school of thought that discourages mirror image practice premised on the belief that certain unilateral features of the form are designed to take into account those energy meridians in the body whose flow of Ch'i is asymmetrical. However it is my belief that the benefits of occasional mirror image practice will far outweigh any possible risks involved.

By practicing in the various fashions described in the exercises above, you will develop adaptive skills and engender a deeper mastery of your own T'ai Chi Ch'uan. By learning how to develop those adaptive skills in the context of knowledge you already have, you will have that process as a model for application throughout your T'ai Chi practice, as well as elsewhere in your life.

DIFFERENT LEARNING STYLES

Another way to optimize your training, or your teaching, is to recognize that there are three distinct primary[1] learning styles, visual, kinesthetic, and audio. Each of us has a primary and a secondary neurological orientation for processing information or various stimuli. The great majority of people are primarily visual learners with either an audio or kinesthetic secondary orientation. What this means is that you will absorb new input better in some ways than in others, and your ability to learn and process information may or may not be different from that of others around you. Just as you tend to absorb information according to your own learning style, so will you tend to express your particular learning style when teaching or communicating, in reflection of your orientation.

Advice for Teachers. [Note: Ostensibly directed toward fellow teachers, by simply reversing the roles, this next section can be apropos to students as well.]

This last point is very important for teachers to recognize. If, for example, you are a visual person who learns best by observing, as a teacher you may unconsciously expect your students to learn by following what you show them to do. Even when giving spoken directions, you may unknowingly express this preference by framing your words in reflection of your own orientation. You may for example, ask others to follow what they see, or what your teaching looks like. Or you may instruct them to follow according to what it sounds like or feels like. For example, "Follow what you see me do." versus, "Follow my spoken directions as I talk you through the move," or, "Try to experience such-and-such a feeling as you practice your move."

It is quite natural for most people to just assume that others share their processing perspective. Your responsibility as a teacher is to share knowledge with others in a way that is meaningful for them. If you fail to accommodate their individual needs, you run the risk of alienating those who learn according to a different style. I once studied with a Sifu who put it succinctly, if crudely. He said, "Teach smart people smart, and stupid people stupid." Despite his apparent lack of politically correct "people skills," he knew how to adjust his teaching style, and was widely regarded as a charismatic leader and an excellent teacher.

As a teacher, the chances are that you have students whose preferred learning style is different from your own preferred teaching style. You may even (unconsciously) hold in higher esteem those students who appear to be apt learners by virtue of their sharing your sensory orientation. This is a very subtle example of what is known as *selective perception.* Consequently, you will need to beware of alienating students who just do not seem to get it the way you teach it.

In an absolute sense, no one learning style is more or less suited than any other style to learning and practicing T'ai Chi. Being a body oriented discipline, T'ai Chi is innately kinesthetic, but visual learners can easily see, or even imagine, themselves at practice (See section on "How to Use the Eyes" in previous chapter on Practice Hints). For visual learners such as these, mirrors and good lighting in your studio can be invaluable assets. While audio learners might seem to be at a slight disadvantage, one's ears are necessarily involved in any form of body discipline requiring balance due to their role in proprioception. None of us uses any one sense to the exclusion of all others. Regardless of someone's processing style, there are ways of addressing the issue to insure that all learning styles are fairly addressed. Remember, each of us has a secondary orientation as a "backup" to the primary.

Flexibility is the Key. One way to address learning discrepancies such as these, is to cover all the bases. In my classes I try to *display* what I am teaching, interwoven with *spoken* directions and *audio* feedback. I also make sure to actually work with people's bodies, *physically adjusting* postures and letting students feel how my own body is positioned (in ways that are appropriate). In this way, students are able to unconsciously translate incoming data to their preferred learning modality. For example, I may suspect someone is a kinesthetic learner if he seems to be having difficulty learning a move which I have shown him repeatedly and with carefully worded directions. In this case, I might actually position his body for him. Or I might adjust my spoken words to address his kinesthetic orientation by asking him to feel or sense the move in a certain way. I might also adjust my visual lead to trigger a kinesthetic response on his part (perhaps by demonstrating, over and over by rote, that which I am teaching while he follows along). If it were the case that the same student was found instead to be an audio learner, I might guide him through the move repeatedly, while cueing him, perhaps in a conspicuously soothing or animated voice, with spoken directions. In this way, his kinesthetic performance would come to be associated with the words and sound of my spoken guidance, and he would likely continue to recall from his memory, consciously or unconsciously, the sound of those words as a means of cueing himself during future solo practice.

The more flexible you are as a teacher in your ability to appeal to a broad range of learning styles, the less likely your students will be to experience frustration or boredom.

If you are a student rather than a teacher, you can take this same advice to heart by paying more conscious attention to cues that intuitively seem to make the most sense to you. You can also take the initiative by consulting your teacher and seeking his or her opinion, advice and/or support on this matter.

How to Determine Your Learning Modality. Close your eyes, and imagine yourself participating in a T'ai Chi class, or any other learning environment. Notice what comes to mind. Do you visualize yourself engaged in practice as if you were watching a video (visual learner), do you recall hearing your teacher's voice guiding you (audio learner), or are you more inclined to feel/sense yourself practicing (kinesthetic learner)? To give you an example of how ingrained and unconscious these orientations can be, I will confess that while writing this last paragraph I caught myself using the phrase, "*running* a video" before changing it to "*watching* a video", thus revealing my own propensity for kinesthetic flavored communication.

I would suggest that you not use the information contained above to govern your training (or teaching) in any global manner, as the learning modalities described may or may not be the final determining factor in how effectively new data is processed. But if you bear this consideration in mind, I am sure you will find that there will be times when it can be gainfully employed to maximize your absorption or conveyance of information, for yourself or for your students.

Notes

1. Non-primary learning styles might include olfactory, gustatory, or extrasensory.

CHAPTER 12

Advanced Rooting Practice and Envelopment Exercises

PULLING TO YOUR ROOT

For more skilled practitioners, a variation to the exercises offered in the earlier chapter on rooting would be to practice them while being pulled rather than pushed. This is quite a bit more challenging because pulling has the apparent effect of separating one away from the earth, whereas pushing tends to reinforce what would seem to be a more natural connection. In T'ai Chi, Pushing and Pulling are generally accorded equal billing. Of course, there is never Yin without Yang, but in my mind, there are clear advantages to pushing versus pulling. If for example, I had to move a stalled car down a flat stretch of road, I would much prefer to push that vehicle rather than pull it. For the same reasons, I would prefer to push rather than pull when dealing with an opponent. It may seem just a matter of semantics, but given the earlier example of two individuals suspended in mid air via ropes, we have already seen how power ultimately stems from the earth. (The only exceptions to this I can think of are isometric forces or muscle contractions such as occur when using weights.)

Generally, the only way you can really pull with any part of your body, is by having something against which you can brace yourself in order to push with another part of your body. By way of example, I happened to be proofing this chapter while away on vacation at the beach. While dragging my beach chair across the sand one morning I realized that in contrast to the disabled car example cited above, I certainly would not want to be pushing my chair across the sand. Pushing in that case, would have proven to be nearly impossible, as my pushing would only have reinforced the connection of the chair to the earth (see Figure 12-1a). Pulling was definitely easier and more natural, but only because I was able to dig in by pushing my feet into the sand as I pulled (see Figure 12-1b). Any action may ostensibly appear to be one of pulling, but below the surface of most pulling forces is a push of one sort or another. Pushing is therefore more efficient and more economical than pulling and, as such, should be your action of choice.

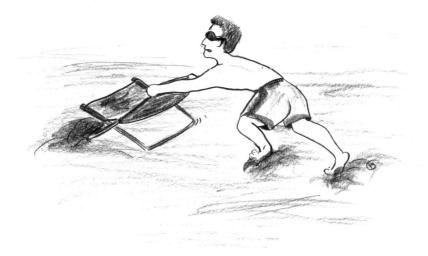

Figure 12-1a. Sometimes a push is a push...

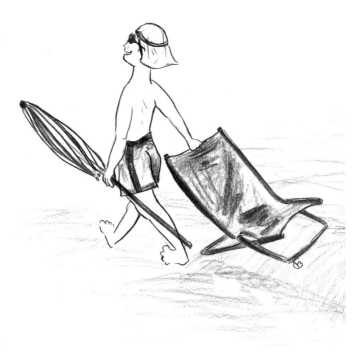

Figure 12-1b. ...and sometimes a push is a pull.

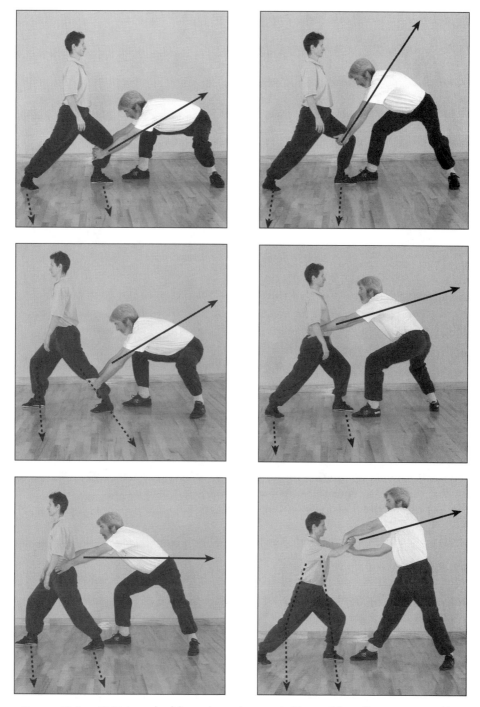

Figures 12-2 to 12-7. In each of these photos the intended force of the Puller is represented by the solid arrow. The redirection of that force into the earth by the subject is represented by the broken arrow.

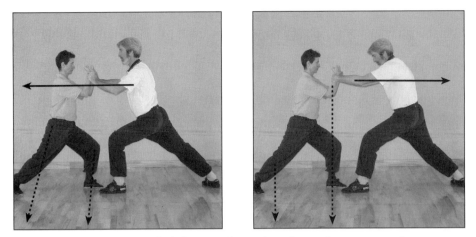

Figures 12-8a, b. The helper can alternately push or pull to encourage the subject to develop adaptive rooting skills.

The basic idea of this two person pulling practice is the same as for the earlier pushing exercise, only instead of your partner pushing to the far foot, he will pull to the near foot. Begin by again imagining yourself rooted from the waist down. Once you are ready, your partner should pull, first at the lower portions of the body, starting with the lower part of the forward leg. Then moving up to the knee, being careful here not to pull lateral to the joint. Then up to the waist, and finally pulling at the torso and the arms. The important thing for you to remember each time your partner exerts a pulling force is to not pull back, rather relax down and redirect the force of his pull, aligning his pull with your skeletal structure, so that it disperses down through your body and into the earth. At that point of dispersion into the earth, you will in effect, be executing a benign, versus overt, push so that the force and strength of his pull is "borrowed" and matched by the force and alignment (but not strength) of your own push.

OTHER STATIONARY VARIATIONS

Variation 1. The next level of skill requires that you be able to adapt variously between a pushing force and a pulling force. As with the earlier exercises, it is important that you start gently and cautiously. If you are the pusher, you can begin by verbally cueing your partner that you are about to change your force from that of a push to that of a pull, or vice versa. You the pushing partner, can secure a hold at the waist, or you can position your arms forward as illustrated (see Figures 12-8a, b). At first the transition for the pushee in negotiating these alternating forces may feel a bit awkward and contrived. With practice, as your partner's compensatory gap in response time between your push and pull narrows, the transition should become smoother to the point that its presence is hardly noticeable. Once you can do this and the next variation well, you will have a decent stationary root.

Variation 2. This exercise is similar to the previous one except that in this scenario, you will alternate your stance, with first one foot forward, then the other. You as the pushee can prearrange for your partner to at first either pull or push, before eventually giving him free reign to alternate between the two forces. Each time you change your stance, try to do so with minimal loss of root. Of course any loss of root resulting from your stance transition will become immediately evident as your partner's force unsteadies you. Start off slowly, taking as much time as you need to reestablish your root after each stance change. Gradually pick up the pace over future practice sessions, until you and your partner can switch quickly and smoothly back and forth from side to side without you losing your balance.

Regardless of whether you opt to practice these rooting skills with pushing or pulling, or pushing and pulling, be sure to work with your partner from a place of advocacy and leave competition to the tournament scene. Or at least wait until you have reached a far more advanced level of skill.

MOVING PRACTICE

Once you feel you have developed a reasonable command and embodiment of these rooting principles in a stationary mode, it is time to take your practice to the next level. The ability to root is only useful insofar as you can apply it practically in your daily life. For most of us, especially those of us doing T'ai Chi, life does not stand still. It is actually relatively easy to get a feel for rooting while standing still. The body is not moving, and consequently with fewer distractions you can confine the fuller focus of your attention to relaxing into your earth connection. Now you can apply these very same principles of rooting to your moving form practice. In fact, you must do so in order to develop real T'ai Chi skill. Everything you have practiced up until this point has merely been preparation for the moving phase. Remember, T'ai Chi is a dynamic experience, a metaphor for life itself—and life is movement.

ROOTING THROUGH YOUR FORM

Now it is time for this tree to take a walk. At first you will likely find it easier to apply the principles we have covered so far to smaller and more manageable sections of whatever form you practice, rather than the form in its entirety. Limit yourself to perhaps just three or four moves as you begin. Then you can use your experience with those first moves as a model for additional moves once you are ready to move on. I will provide some pointers here, but rather than trying to address a whole range of moves, I will limit my guidance here to the context of simple forward walking. By so doing we can avoid any confusion due to idiosyncrasies between different forms or teachers. Even if you have not yet learned a form, feel free to try the following exercise. Be advised though, there are a lot of details and minutia here, so take it slowly, and do not become frustrated if you are not able to get it all right the first time through. If you are newer at this you will probably find it helpful to refer to the glossary of terms at the back of the book.

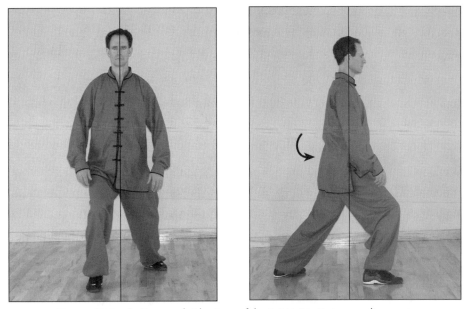

Figures 12-9a, b. Front and side views of the Bai Hui to Perineum alignment.

STEP BY STEP

Begin by standing with your left foot to the front, left knee bent forward and over, but not beyond, the toes below. The left foot should point directly ahead while the back leg is kept straight, its foot angled forty-five degrees[1] or so outward. The distance between your feet should be approximately three 'foot' lengths.

Before you begin to move forward, feel yourself rooted in place just as you did with the earlier stationary practices. Check to see that your *Ba Hui* (crown point) and *Hui Yin* (perineum) are in line and plumb, and that your coccyx is curled slightly under (see Figures 12-9a, b).

Now, press down into the Bubbling Well point of your front foot in order to sink just a wee bit backward into your tailbone. Do this without rising up, and sink back only just far enough so as to release some of the weight from the front of your forward foot. As you begin this movement, you can imagine that your partner is right there before you, hands on your waist, ready to push or pull. This will serve as an incentive to stay rooted and not bounce up.

Now, with your forward foot less fully weighted and the toes raised off the ground, turn your front toes out to the side (thirty to forty-five degrees) in preparation to shift forward (see Figures 12-10a, b). Pay attention as you do so, even before putting the toes back down, to the left and right sides of the Qua (inguinal crease). Having flared your left toes out, you should now have the feeling that your left Qua has been peeled slightly open. Beware as your left Qua opens, of any tendency for your opposite (right) Qua to (incorrectly) collapse toward your center. Maintaining both sides of your Qua open will require your conscientious

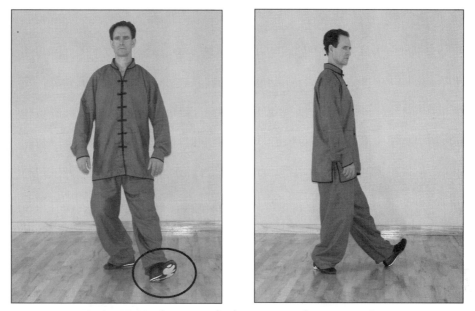

Figures 12-10a, b. Front and side views. Note front toe turned out.

attention, and may at first take some getting used to. The importance of keeping both Qua open should not be underestimated. This is what will enable you to maintain your root in any transition from one posture to the next.

Next roll your left foot down and flat, as if it were a front-wheel-driven tire, its tread grabbing the road to pull its load forward. As your left foot flattens down it will begin to pull its own knee along with it. As this happens you should, simultaneously, have a feeling at the base of your spine of your tailbone curling under. Feel your tailbone as if it were connected to the front foot and pressing your entire body forward as one solid unit (see Figures 12-11a, b).

Once your forward foot is fully flat continue bending your front knee, being careful to maintain its alignment directly over the foot below, versus collapsing it outward or inward. Again you must be attentive to maintain both Qua open. Shift forward until the front knee is over the foot below and the back leg has become fully straight.

Continue driving your weight forward from the tailbone, allowing the back (right) foot to lift up from its heel, as if it were a suction cup being peeled from the floor (see Figure 12-12). If you have managed to keep the Qua properly open, you will now be able to move the right knee smoothly forward and through to the front, without any rising up or bouncing to undermine your stability.

As your now-forward right leg reaches full extension try to extend the toes just a bit further before touching the heel down. As the right heel reaches for the floor feel it extending away from the tailbone (see Figures 12-13 & 12-14). Once your heel contacts the floor, roll your right foot down flat as if now it is the front-

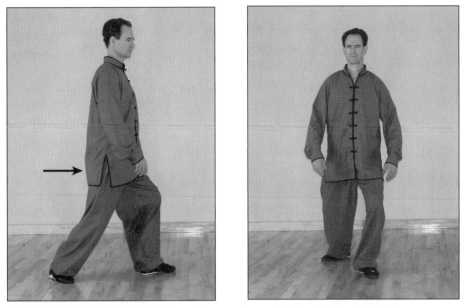

Figure 12-11a, b. Front & side views. Notice the front foot turned out in preparation to advance. Tailbone presses the body forward.

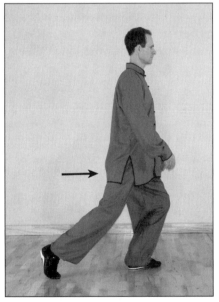

Figure 12-12. Tailbone continues pressing forward as the back heel peels up.

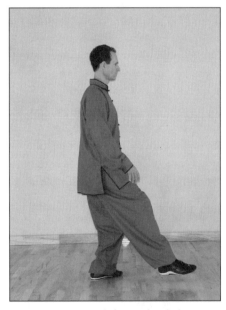

Figure 12-13. Reach forward with the toe...

wheel-driven tire. As you are doing this, press down into the Bubbling Well point of the left foot (now in back) and use that force to drive the sacrum/tailbone (along with the rest of the body) forward to complete one step.

Having this single step now as a model, you can proceed to practice your T'ai Chi stepping on the other side, and so on. When you move like this in T'ai Chi, you will feel like a tractor, slow, steady, and sure.

The directions for the previous exercise are designed not only to guide you in the intricacies of correct stepping, but also to give you some idea of the quality of attention and the level of detail necessary in order to develop your T'ai Chi overall, to a high level of proficiency.

ADVANCED FORM PRACTICE

Once you feel as if you are able to maintain a well-rooted connection, yet remain soft and fluid while practicing the form, you can arrange for your part-

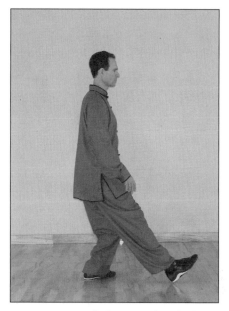

Figure 12-14. ...before extending the heel to reconnect to the earth.

ner to assist you by pushing at first, then pulling, and eventually pushing and/or pulling as you flow from posture to posture.

At this stage your partner need only apply occasional pushes to spot check the quality of your root, or for a more demanding challenge, he can lean in (or out) while holding on to you, thus providing a constant burden or drag on your movements (see Figure 12-15). Of course both of you will have to agree on how much resistance is to be applied lest it become onerous and counterproductive. Ideally, you should be able to proceed through your form as if you were barely even aware

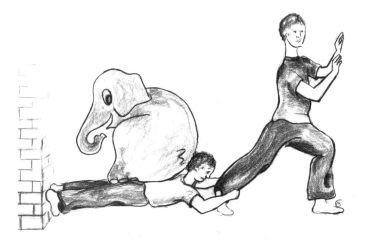

Figure 12-15. When you've got your root, ain't nothin' gonna stop you.

of your partner's presence, let alone his efforts to reveal any flaws in the quality and consistency of your root.

ADVANCED ENVELOPMENT EXERCISES

Note: the following exercises are geared toward more experienced practitioners.

Easy Does It At First. Try this with a partner. As is usually the case with two person exercises, you will want to begin by getting a feel for the drill without the added challenge of working at cross-purposes with your partner. Position yourself in a well-rooted stance and have your partner place one of his hands on your chest or abdominal area. Your partner can slowly and gently begin to lean in with a bit of weight. In contrast to the earlier rooting exercise in which you held more firmly structured while transferring your partner's force down to the earth, in this exercise you will relax to become insubstantial, softening and yielding to melt before your partner's force, even as you maintain your root. As your partner continues to simply lean his weight into you, feel in your own body where you can absorb and envelop his force without actually becoming burdened by it. Your partner meanwhile, benefits from this by exploring how his displacing touch elicits your yielding envelopment. Once you have developed a reasonable command of this you can proceed to the next level.

Hide and Seek. In this variation of the earlier practice you and your partner will be slightly less collaborative. Here you will begin as before with your partner placing his hand on your chest or abdomen. This time your partner will begin using his touch to slowly seek out

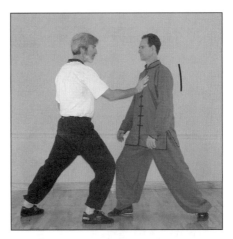

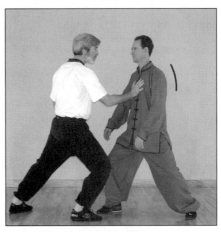

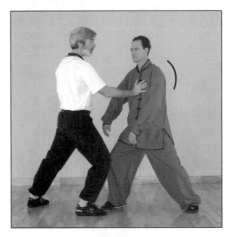

Figures 12-16a, b, c. Yield to your opponent's attack, luring him in.

your center with the idea in mind of moving you off from your place of balance and rootedness. For you the challenge will be to yield and elude in a manner that does not allow your partner to "lock on" to your center. For both of you, "success" will require your using the aforementioned *Ting Jing* listening skill in order to remain sensitive to the other's whereabouts and intention.

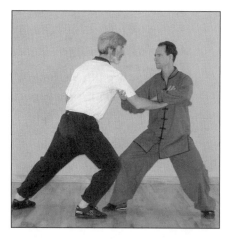

In your case, you want to "trick" your partner, luring him in to over commit, until you have him right where you want him (see Figures 12-16a, b, c). Think of wrapping around his force, but without letting it in quite so deep that you are left without an escape route. The more deeply you are able to envelop your partner's force, the more likely he will find himself caught beyond the point of no return. By the time he realizes his mistake, he will have been enveloped too deeply in your own territory to be able to extricate himself. At this point, you can either "disappear", or turn the tables to issue a displacing force of your own (see Figures 12-16 d, e, f).

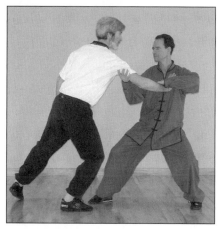

This of course, is a training exercise. If your partner's punch were real, you would not allow him to penetrate so deeply into your space. This practice approach will enable you to safely develop an enhanced sensitivity for establishing your own comfortable parameters in preparation for any incoming force. On the surface, the previous exercises could amount to little more than freestyle pushing hands competition. What distinguishes them from competition, is the de-emphasis on goal/winning with the focus rather on actualizing the principles of displacement and envelopment.

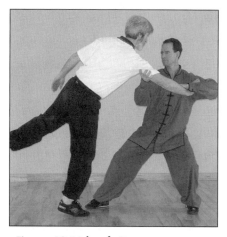

Figures 12-16d, e, f. Once your opponent is overextended you can borrow his force to turn the tables.

137

Notes

1. A word here on angles and the geometry of your form. The exact angles of your feet in relationship to each other may vary somewhat at any given point, and from person to person according to your own physiology. Some styles may emphasize postures or positions in apparent contrast to the specifics of the exercise described. Do not despair, as the principles, if not the exact angles, are universally valid. The angles may merely need to be "tweaked" for application in other styles.

CHAPTER 13

Where to Go From Here, A Consumer's Guide

So now you are interested in pursuing a study of T'ai Chi? Where do you go from here? The first thing that I recommend is that you take some time to reflect and ask yourself what exactly is it that prompts your interest in T'ai Chi. In what way or ways are you hoping to benefit from any studies you undertake? Your personal agenda may include any of the following: mind/body exercise, "spiritual" movement, whole body exercise, fun and novel activity, getting in shape, doctor referral, flexibility, stress reduction, self-defense, "don't know, but it sounds cool," etc. The clearer you can be with yourself about your priorities, the greater the likelihood that you will be able to find an instructor or school that matches your agenda. Be as clear as you can with yourself, but do not be close-minded. The benefits of T'ai Chi are myriad and they will likely, extend beyond your own agenda.

VARIABLES TO CONSIDER AND RESOURCES TO ACCESS

Your choice of schools will probably be strongly influenced by your location. If you are in an urban area, there may be several schools from which to choose. If you live out in the country, your choices may be more limited. If you simply lack access to a school you can try reading books on the subject or viewing videos. These may teach you something about T'ai Chi but remember, there is no substitute for direct experience with a credible teacher.

As with anything else, it is always a good idea to check with friends for recommendations. The phone book may also provide some leads. If the Yellow Pages do not show any listings for T'ai Chi schools in your area, call any Kung Fu or Karate schools listed to see if they might provide a referral. Sometimes classes can be found at local colleges, senior centers, community centers, or wellness organizations. In warmer climates some teachers eschew indoor facilities in favor of the local park. Bear in mind, because of low overhead, these classes are less likely to advertise in the phone book. If you are someone who teaches or already studies another form of martial arts, another possibility is to consider arranging to host a teacher from outside your area for workshops or seminars at your school. Many of the better teachers in this country travel far and wide to share their knowledge in just this way. You can also locate schools or find out about other people's seminars by checking out trade magazines such as *T'ai Chi* or *Taijiquan Journal* (See References).

MAKING CONTACT

Once you have found a school or schools, call ahead to inquire about the basics: scheduling, location, class times, parking, costs, etc. Then ask if it would be possible to visit the school for an appointment with the instructor, perhaps before a scheduled class. The instructor will probably want to know what prompts your interest, and you should ask the instructor to share any relevant information on his or her background of studies and on his or her teaching philosophy. Ask the instructor how long (s)he has been involved practicing/teaching T'ai Chi or other martial arts? Does (s)he maintain any affiliation with other organizations or teachers? Has (s)he any adjunctive professional credentials? It is not unusual to find T'ai Chi teachers who have a background in other service areas such as acupuncture or academia. This may be a plus to the extent that good service or teaching skills in one area may carry over into their T'ai Chi teaching method. The instructor's lineage may or may not be revealing of his or her practice or teaching skill, but having read this book, you should have some basis for determining any instructor's basic credibility. I would caution you to beware of false claims of affiliation. I have known of instructors who took a single class or perhaps a seminar with some recognized T'ai Chi master and then advertised their "affiliation" to falsely inflate their credentials. Finally, be sure to ask about the martial content of the classes. Do students learn Pushing Hands or weapons, and at what point in your training can this be expected to occur?

GOOD COMMUNICATION IS ESSENTIAL

During this first visit, you will want to register the actual information the instructor is sharing, plus get an *intuitive* sense of the teacher and the school. Ask yourself if rapport is likely to develop. It is reasonable for you to expect fairly direct answers to reasonable questions. Do not settle for any mystical mumbo jumbo. If clear communication is not forthcoming now, how realistic can be any expectations that it will improve later on? Remember, you are about to enter into a new learning environment where clear communication with your instructor will likely be the most critical factor in determining how fully you benefit from your studies. Use this opportunity to disclose any special considerations you may have in terms of your agenda, personal concerns/goals, including any pertinent medical information. Before enrolling, you should want to get a sense that you can comfortably entrust yourself to a teacher's guidance, and that your best interests will be taken to heart.

CHECK IT OUT, ASK QUESTIONS

Be sure to sit in and observe an actual class in progress prior to committing yourself for any program of study. Get a feel for the physical space. Notice details such as the size of the classes, the gender composition, and the age range. Ask if the class you are watching is representative of an average class, or if it is in any way atypical. Remember, T'ai Chi can be quite a broad and deep learning process with an emphasis that varies from class to class. Ask how experienced are the students in the class? Are there separate classes available for beginners and for more advanced students so as to meet your developing needs as you gain more experience? As you watch, try to imagine yourself actually participating in the class. Bear in mind however, that any new learning can seem intimidating at first to a casual observer.

Notice how the instructor and/or any teaching assistants interact with the students. Do students receive personal attention? Do the instructors provide guidance tailored to the class? Is that guidance visual, spoken, kinesthetic (hands on)? Is the class structured in an organized fashion (very organized, loosely organized?)? Are the students required to wear uniforms? Some schools require uniforms and some do not. T'ai Chi classes generally tend to be a bit looser and less formal than external style classes, but martial arts style workout pants and a school T-shirt may be standard issue. One thing I have never heard of any credible T'ai Chi school doing is employing belts for ranking as is done in Karate systems. If the opportunity presents itself, and it does not distract ongoing classes in progress, it might be a good idea to introduce yourself to any of the already active students, before or after a class, to see if you can get some sense of the school's social environment. Ask other students how they feel about the school and what benefits they feel they have derived from their participation.

COMMITTING TO A COURSE OF STUDY

Once you have made a decision to participate in classes, you will need to address the issue of commitment, both the commitment you are willing to make, as well as any that the school may ask from you as a matter of policy. Some schools will charge a simple monthly tuition, others may ask that you commit for a period of three or six months, or even a year. You need to bear in mind that T'ai Chi will take time and effort to learn and that in order to derive the sought after benefits you will need to stick with your practice. One or two months are barely enough time to get your feet wet, let alone achieve any real proficiency. I recommend, providing you are comfortable with the school and the teacher, that you plan on a six to twelve month trial commitment to give T'ai Chi a chance to work its magic for you. It generally takes about a year for students to learn the 108 movement *Yang* form, but that can vary widely according to the teacher and the style or form taught. Of course learning the moves is just a first step. Remember that T'ai Chi is as much a process as it is a goal. You can spend a lifetime engaged in developing its mastery. Do not sell yourself short by limiting your horizons.

PART 3

PERSONAL ACCOUNTS, LECTURE TRANSCRIPTS/ MUSINGS AND APPENDICES

CHAPTER 14

Stories

T'ai Chi
To be lost in the clouds of my mind.
To walk though my body, with my body.
To touch my soul, with my soul.
Such are the dreams of a young and foolish man
who knows not of the futileness of life,
and believes he can love dewdrops,
and hold butterflies in the skies
of his own mind.
The simple way you teach us,
guide us with the shadow of your hand.
The way you let us teach ourselves, experience and comprehend.
We long to feel the air breathe us,
to live without explaining why.
To throw away the secret chains that bind us,
to have a chance to try.
We love you for your understanding, we want to be like you.
To feel the essence of our heart's spirit.
to make our bodies new.
      —Richard, 1975

The poem above was written for me by one of my T'ai Chi students back in 1975 when I was just a fledgling teacher. Throughout the years this poem has served as an inspiration for me and as a touching reminder that as a T'ai Chi teacher I can have a lasting and powerful impact on the lives of those I teach. Of course the reverse is true as well. If it was not for my students I could not have been a teacher. One of the many important lessons I have learned over the years is that each and every student has a story of his or her own that sets him or her uniquely apart from all others. Yet there are often common and recurring threads in the collective T'ai Chi experience. I would like to use this chapter to share with you the T'ai Chi experiences, in their own words, of some of my students. I believe that just as I have been inspired by my student Richard's poem, in a way that he probably never imagined possible or even likely, you may find some inspiration or validation in relating to the T'ai Chi experiences and personal accounts that follow. The contributing students are identified by gender and age only, and their stories have been presented in their own words with a minimum of editing.

Female, age 37. T'ai Chi first presented itself to me in the form of a book. I was looking in one of my favorite haunts, a large bookstore, perusing through volumes in the "Eastern Philosophy/Martial Arts" section, when fate put the book *"T'ai Chi Classics"* by Waysun Liao into my hands. The few paragraphs I spot-read in the store were promising, so I brought the book home and worked my way through it. What a revelation! This was exactly what I had been looking for! I do believe strongly in the power of the mind. The explanations given in Mr. Liao's book about cultivating Ch'i, and ultimately developing Jing, were enough to convince me that T'ai Chi was "The Way" I needed to go if I hoped to really develop the capabilities I desired.

The next day I browsed the local phone book for schools offering T'ai Chi courses. I found a school practically next door to where I live, offering comprehensive classes including: form practice, stretching, breathing exercises, rooting exercises, sensitivity training for push-hands practice, and an opportunity to learn about and discuss the philosophy underlying T'ai Chi. Sifu is always ready to give the reasons for certain moves or exercises, and to explain the thought behind the external form. He does not however, serve up insights on demand. By providing just enough information to stimulate the thought process, he rather lets us find our own truths in the teachings. If questions arise, I discovered that I do not need to ask them immediately—if I just continue to observe and pay close attention to what is being taught, answers will almost always present themselves over the course of the next few classes.

Even though I very much enjoyed the challenge of learning something completely new, the first few months proved to be difficult. Being the newcomer, I felt a lot like the "odd person out". Besides my being a stranger in what appeared to be a closely-knit group, everybody else seemed to know exactly what they were doing. They moved gracefully through the form, while I was craning my neck and tying knots into my spine and extremities to follow Sifu, only to forget most of the moves as soon as I was back home again. To say that I became frustrated after a while would be an understatement. I am not an outgoing person, and to "face the crowd" at class, feeling awkward and pretty stupid with my clumsy moves, at times took more courage than I could muster. But forcing myself to make it through this phase and not give up and drop out also helped improve my discipline and strengthened the resolve that after all, I was doing this to better myself, not to impress other people or gain their acceptance.

Then, imperceptibly at first, the form settled in, and I found that I could repeat most of the first section at home without getting stuck every few seconds. Was I proud of myself! Slowly, I came to feel less embarrassed when singled out for correction of my form or for demonstration of a certain move.

Interestingly enough, for T'ai Chi I had to unlearn a lot of what had been ingrained over the years: turn the foot in rather than out as demanded in ballet,

let the shoulders sag a little and round them to achieve the concave chest, and tuck in the tailbone, instead of standing ramrod straight in military fashion. After a year of practice I have yet to master all that. My shoulders still secretly hunch up on me, and my behind stubbornly sticks out like a sore thumb! But as my body perception sharpens, these faults diminish—I hope.

The part I still find hardest to comprehend and learn is how to be totally relaxed while still retaining enough tension to execute the moves gracefully and with power. One prime example would be the opening, basic stance: it is necessary to be rooted, which, as far as I understand, is supposed to include a feeling of tension going from one foot up the leg and then down the other leg to the other foot, as if both feet grab the ground and pull together, while all the time maintaining the *open Qua*—but how can I be relaxed and tense at the same time? It's the same with extending my arms in the single whip position—if I extend my arms as far as I can (with the shoulders DOWN!!!) and sink as well as possible, trying to maintain a well-rooted stance, I am NOT relaxed at all! These are only some of the many things I am struggling with, but I presume that with time and patience I will one day gain the insight of how to apply the principles correctly.

I find that T'ai Chi is teaching me to move more economically, particularly noticeable when I am out lobstering and hoisting traps. I attempt to sink the center, move from the waist and let the skeletal frame rather than the muscles carry the moves through and do the work. My success at this pays off with rewards such as a lot less fatigue and fewer backaches.

T'ai Chi is also helping me to learn to observe and feel my body "from the inside out", so to speak. It has become easier to take the proverbial step back when I realize that I am "in too deep", i.e. my shoulders are hunched, my neck muscles tighten, and my breathing becomes shallow and erratic. I can then attempt to remedy these situations by either finding a quiet spot and going through part of the form, or if a quiet spot is nowhere to be found, by just sitting still, breathing deeply, calming my mind and body, and mentally performing the T'ai Chi moves. Afterwards, I am usually able to address persistent problems in a much calmer fashion.

Another positive development is a remarkable absence of those annoying little aches and pains and seasonal colds that used to take their toll at least once every few months!

Add to that the feeling of triumphal achievement when I finally have the externals of yet another move "down pat", and the challenge of then starting the real work of tackling the internals of those same moves, and I have a combination that makes T'ai Chi ever interesting, never boring.

As to the spiritual aspect: T'ai Chi, and in particular the philosophy of Taoism, are teaching me how to find and travel on the path towards serenity and connectedness to all........ well, call it "creation". To use a fashionable expression, "I am shifting my paradigm". What was important before, e.g. career and money, relationships in the sense of acceptance by others and recognition, material possessions—these have taken a back seat to goals such as inner peace, understanding, and non-judgmental acceptance of everything around me, living or inanimate (and who's to say what is and what is not?).

I also find that the non-verbal connection I have to certain people in my life has strengthened and that I am beginning to be able to discern and control where before I had to simply experience and accept.

Learning about Taoist ideals and practicing T'ai Chi and meditation help me overcome, and in certain instances banish altogether, periods of anxiety or worry about the future. By finding my own center, both physically and spiritually, and then branching out, I become aware of the fact that I am but an infinitesimal part of this universe, and that revelation prevents me from being caught up and becoming mired in the quicksand of petty day-to-day trials and tribulations. I allow them less and less to have any lasting effect on my life.

This does not mean that I just sail through life unaffected by anything, ever happy and blissful. Developing the state of existence I desire is a continuous process with ups and downs. Sometimes I attain the serenity I am looking for, other times I fall back into the old groove of letting myself become drawn in, overwhelmed, and brought down. But at least now I know what I want to achieve and the way to go about it, so all it takes is a conscious effort, at the point of realization, to retreat and extricate myself.

My ultimate goal? To become a person resting in herself, connected to the Tao, with knowledge and abilities enabling me to help people in need of physical or spiritual assistance and guidance, and to thus do my part in working towards a unified, peaceful world on Earth. I do believe that in Taoism and T'ai Chi I have finally found what I have been looking for ever since I can remember, the means to achieve this goal. I know I have a long, long way to go, but then, I have the rest of my life for this journey!

Author's notes: This person is someone who is very clearly in touch with her own process. She knew just what she was looking for before she found it in T'ai Chi. That she committed herself to the process and discipline of study despite the challenges of being a somewhat shy newcomer in an unfamiliar environment evidences a well-developed capacity for delayed gratification. Finally, she has a clear sense of goal in terms of how she plans to use her T'ai Chi training to fulfill her own personal agenda over time.

Female, age 50. My journey in T'ai Chi began seven years ago through what, at the time, seemed an accidental convolution of events, events which in retrospect seem to have been prophetic.

Three components of what has evolved for me into a lifetime journey converged in one place, at one time. The setting was my chiropractor's office and the elements were my introspection on the many physical problems I was having at the relatively young age of 43, an escalating cholesterol level then reading at 267, and the presence in the same room of a young man wearing a T-shirt emblazoned with the words "Kung Fu/ T'ai Chi/ Internal Arts."

The T-shirt sparked my memory of articles I had read during my undergraduate studies that had equated one hour of T'ai Chi practice to one hour of good psychotherapy. Before leaving the office that day I made the decision to immerse myself in a study of T'ai Chi.

This decision was in no small way influenced by a lifetime of high heel shoes (the fashion mandate of my profession), combined with the long term effects of high impact aerobics, racquetball, and running on hard pavement. Outwardly I appeared to be in "tip top" shape, 5'2", 110 pounds, tanned, and toned. But inwardly, I suffered intense back pain which produced sleepless nights, bunions from the heels for which my podiatrist was considering surgery, an all-time energy low, and at the conclusion of my chiropractic visit that day a diagnosis of osteoarthritis in my neck plus a mild scoliosis. I was a skeletal wreck!

Outwardly, my life had been progressing quite positively. I had just earned my B.A. in Psychology and was about to embark on a Master's program. However the contrast between outward fulfillment on a day-to-day basis and my sleepless nights of physical pain were just too incongruent to ignore.

That was before my T'ai Chi journey began all those years ago. My tentative first attempts at the T'ai Chi form, as a novice under my Sifu, allowed me to evolve eventually in my practice to the point that I now conduct my own T'ai Chi classes. As I teach, I continue to learn and heal myself along with my students. As a professional caregiver I have found that in truly caring for myself, the quality of care I provide others is enhanced.

Today, my cholesterol is 188, my back and neck pain is minimal, and my orthodic foot supports reside where they belong, in my sock drawer. Though my professional schedule is more demanding now than ever before, I can always take time for T'ai Chi, using my breathing skills to feel more at one with myself.

Author's notes: This student's initial exposure to T'ai Chi (at her chiropractor's office) underscores both the importance and the increasing frequency of interdisciplinary referrals via other health care practitioners. (Though not referenced in her personal account, her D.C. has referred several students my way.) I regard individuals who are already oriented toward person-centered health care modalities as likely candidates for T'ai Chi Ch'uan. This person's account also speaks to the relevance of T'ai Chi in addressing life-style based stress issues whether objective, as is the case with cholesterol or blood pressure, or subjective as with pain or anxiety. Finally, her account emphasizes the importance and benefits of health care providers attending to their own needs in order to stay balanced within.

Male, age 71. At age seventy-one it isn't easy to keep good health, but I believe exercise helps, and T'ai Chi has solved that problem for me. At each class Sifu incorporates a lesson theme into our class time, "rooting", or "uprooting", or "moving from the waist", etc. It seems endless, with some new material to learn or a new way of looking at things in every class.

I had actually taken a bit of T'ai Chi years ago and only recently resumed my practice. Being retired, I didn't want to just laze around the house, so I took up activities like biking, walking, and swimming. But I still felt something was missing, so I took up T'ai Chi again. The T'ai Chi really works both my mind and my body, leaving me feeling refreshed and energized after each work out. After just a few months of being back in class I feel my muscles are more relaxed and I can bend with greater flexibility. When I have spare time at home I practice the form and am starting to remember the moves. I feel that T'ai Chi has helped me a lot and I plan to keep up my practice.

Author's notes: Older students can derive tremendous benefit and pleasure simply by recapturing some of the energy, and freedom from physical limitations, that characterized the days of their youth. Increased flexibility (or even simply a moratorium on the decline of flexibility) plus the acquisition of new skills can lend new meaning to the lives of those beyond their physical prime.

Male, age 16. When I first began learning martial arts I was not studying T'ai Chi, but Kung Fu. At that point I had trouble getting the techniques down correctly, since I was only six years old and I hadn't yet fully developed all my motor skills. I then drifted away from practicing at the age of 8, and started again when I was around 11 years old. After that I had on and off again lessons in Kung Fu empty hand forms and weapons.

In fact, it wasn't until a year ago, that I wanted to understand more about other forms of martial arts. So I asked my dad if we both could sign up for T'ai Chi Ch'uan. I did not quite know what to expect, partially because I wasn't too successful keeping up with Kung Fu when I was younger, but I am very glad to have studied T'ai Chi under my Sifu. He was very good at teaching me, and I immediately got incredibly interested in T'ai Chi and Ch'i Kung.

I have been so interested that I bought many books to use as textbooks in order to help me further my skills. After only a year of learning under Sifu, I have already boosted my self-confidence. I have learned about Ch'i flow, skeletal structuring, muscular efficiency, and the human aging cycle. This is much more than I thought I would ever learn to say the least. I still want to continue the development of my skills and I want to keep learning. It has become so important in my day-to-day routine that I don't know what I would do without its lessons.

Author's notes: This teenager presents as uncharacteristically non-egocentric for a youngster in mid-adolescence. In my mind his account provides a compelling argument for the presentation of T'ai Chi as a "living philosophy" to young adults.

Male, age 44. My story began back in the early 1980's when a friend recommended that I take up a study of *Pa Qua Chang*. After doing a bit of research and asking some questions it became obvious that I was not going to find a *Pa Qua* teacher convenient to where I lived. However the yellow pages confirmed that there were plenty of martial arts schools locally. I began to call around to them, finally settling on one in the town next to where I lived. Although the main focus of the school and the instructor was on Kung Fu, T'ai Chi was also part of the curriculum and gave me a place to start. At that point just getting started was the most important thing to me.

I started by taking classes weekly and it soon became obvious to me that this art, although appearing very simple, had much more depth than I'd anticipated. I had played many different sports as a youth and young adult, but none of them prepared me for the workout that my body was getting from T'ai Chi, both during warm up exercises and during the actual learning of the movements of the form. The practice wasn't particularly strenuous in terms of exertion, yet it was challenging on many levels. Muscles that I never knew I had made themselves known to me. I hurt in places that I didn't know could hurt. Old sports injuries came out of hiding and reminded me of my youthful indiscretions. I would like to say that it was a good hurt that I was feeling, but that would be untrue. In spite of being reminded by my Sifu to go only as far as I felt comfortable, I pushed beyond those limits whenever I could. So began my journey, limping and groaning and wondering just what I had gotten myself into.

The first hurdle I came to in the study of T'ai Chi was the number of moves in the form. It was no simple feat learning each and being able to do them so that they had some resemblance to my Sifu's demonstration of them. I had to put aside even thinking about the internal side of T'ai Chi in order to concentrate on the physical challenge of learning the sequence of the moves. Apparently I had given my initial presumed intellectual understanding of T'ai Chi far too much weight in the big picture. While learning the form it became abundantly clear to me that until I had the moves and their sequence down, I would not be able to begin work on any of the deeper aspects of the practice that I had read about and aspired to. So I concentrated on learning the sequence until I could do it without having to search my memory for what move came next.

It wasn't long before simple practice of the form, without even considering any of the underlying principles, began to reap its own benefits. My back problems, a constant source of pain for me, hurt less during the day. My knees, which were battered from old sports injuries and prone to painfully "going out" on me during the simplest of everyday movements, seemed to be strengthening and stabilizing, causing me fewer and fewer problems as my form work progressed. I began to feel more balance in my step, my form, my demeanor, and my life in general. I found that my practice had a calming effect on me, a feeling I began to want with me all the time, not just when doing my form practice. I was already culling benefits from my T'ai Chi practice knowing full well that I had barely scratched the surface of what the art had to offer. I felt I was ready to move on to the next step. Little did I know that the staircase I was climbing reached out of my sight and that over the next fifteen years I would take many such steps, each building on the knowledge and understanding of the step that had come before it.

I consider myself very lucky to have had the same Sifu under whom I have studied over the past fifteen years. It's not that I consider his personal knowledge of T'ai Chi to be boundless, or even that I think he is that gifted a teacher of the art. What keeps me coming back is his understanding of the many facets of T'ai Chi, the incredible depth of the art, and his ability to work with and advance the place that any particular student is at in their study. He recognizes that he too is a student, constantly learning and improving his expression of the art. I have observed that his own understanding of all the subtleties of T'ai Chi has increased dramatically over the years I have studied under him. I too am a beneficiary of his learning.

Over the years of my studies there have been many instances, mostly by way of work peripheral to the direct practice of T'ai Chi, that have directly impacted my understanding of the art. Sometimes the best path to a clear understanding of a concept is an indirect route, and that has surely been the case with me. Through workshops not related specifically to T'ai Chi, but rather to complementary, underlying, or supporting principles, I've had flashes of insight into aspects of my own form practice that were previously lacking. Upon grasping a better understanding of any one of the complexities that underlies this wonderful art, it is both humbling and invigorating to come to grips with how clueless I had been.

Any time that I have felt a deeper understanding of one level of T'ai Chi, I have made it my business to again recognize the flight of stairs I am climbing as I learn. The new recognition is but another step in my understanding of the complexities of the art. At each one of these milestones I feel like I am a beginner all over again, trying to integrate my new awareness into all that I have learned before it. It is a kind of breaking down and rebuilding process, getting back to the essential basics of what it is that I think I know about T'ai Chi and then taking the new understanding I have and trying to make it a part of my form. I have begun to appreciate the calm and blissful look of the people in the parks practicing T'ai Chi at whatever level they are at, seemingly content to always be a beginner with so much more to learn about this simple and elegant art form.

I cannot possibly describe all the areas of my life that my T'ai Chi practice has affected. A person who knew me fifteen years ago would probably not recognize the new me inside. For me T'ai Chi has truly been an internal art. Each aspect of T'ai Chi that I have studied has become a part of my persona. The balance in my form has translated to more balance in my life. The rootedness and centering I feel in my form practice have also spilled over into my personal life, giving me a quiet confidence. There is a calm and deliberate sense of vitality that has also carried over into my waking hours. I would guess the single most notable result of my study of T'ai Chi is my being less destination oriented. I find that I enjoy the journey much more than the arrival at any particular place, making me more spontaneous and aware of my surroundings. The blinders are off, as it were. This was never my goal, but rather a wonderful by-product of my studies..

In the time that I have studied T'ai Chi, life's events and challenges have pulled me away from taking formal classes from time to time for one reason or another, sometimes for long periods. During these times I have kept up with at least some of the basic practices as a means of staying connected to the benefits I have felt from T'ai Chi. Each time that the challenge at hand has passed, I have found myself drawn back to the formal school setting, enjoying the group energy and the feedback that the class dynamic brings to my practice. It is at these times especially that I can recognize how much I have to learn about T'ai Chi. I see my studies as being a lifelong pursuit with no particular goal in mind other than to learn as much as I can about the subtle nature and complexities of T'ai Chi. The assimilation and integration at each step reaches way beyond the classroom setting and form practice and has become a very tangible part of who I am. This realization makes me happy and grateful that I took that first step.

Author's notes: Again, as with the first account, this individual has clearly benefited from the evolving process of T'ai Chi as a presence in his life over a number of years. His account also illustrates how easy it can be to think you know something, until you get to the next level of knowledge, only to realize you didn't know quite as much as you thought you did. In the same way, the manner in which T'ai Chi effects us in our lives can be fluid, varying according to whatever else might be going on in our lives at any given time.

Male, age 45. I began my studies of T'ai Chi about a year ago. I started T'ai Chi with the hope that it would help to relieve my stress level. Whenever I'm under a great deal of stress, my body's response is to tense up in my shoulders and lower back, which leads to chronic pain. Since starting at T'ai Chi, I feel as if I am able to identify when tension is building up in my body before it becomes a problem, and then signal myself to focus on my breathing and relax those areas where tension usually happens.

Another benefit is that my focusing has improved markedly since I started with T'ai Chi. My mind used to get to the point that it would bounce around like a dropped super ball, going this way and that way, out of control. But T'ai Chi affects me like a meditation that grounds me and centers my thoughts. My emotions also, seem to be in a more stable flow now. Because of this I'm less prone to impulsivity and less likely to make stupid mistakes under volatile conditions.

I've noticed changes in my body as well. My balance has increased and my overall physical fitness has improved. I now have the endurance to stay in certain positions for prolonged periods, as well as being more able to move quickly for self-defensive purposes. I feel I still a have a ways to go in both these areas, but I credit my overall personal improvement to the slow motion moves of my T'ai Chi and my related Ch'i Kung practices. I am quite pleased with my T'ai Chi training and I fully expect to continue with this discipline for the rest of my life. T'ai Chi really doesn't require a lot of time each day, but it does require a consistent effort. I am proud to say I am a T'ai Chi student.

Author's notes: This student continues to move in and out of T'ai Chi according to the volatility in his life, which he hinted at in the account above. The question here for me as a teacher is, how can I provide my student guidance in T'ai Chi as a useful tool to mitigate that volatility and yet remain appreciative, respectful and supportive, versus intrusive, amidst the current realities of his life?

Female, age 47. I must be at that period some of us reach in our lives when we look back, and perhaps realize that we want to continue on a path left years ago, or that we need to take a risk to fulfill our desire for accomplishment. In my case this seems somehow exacerbated by my recent discovery, through independent testing, of my own unique learning disorder issues, not quite ADD, but "slow visual processing along with extreme attention to detail", yet "very good attention when rules are clear." I actually view my detail-oriented style as an asset in my work as an editor, as well as in my being a T'ai Chi student. It's become clear to me that I can learn what I want to learn if only I seek out the way of learning that is best for me.

My interest in T'ai Chi began as a result of hanging around the school to occasionally observe my son's Kung Fu classes. While perusing some flyers on T'ai Chi, the idea of "being in the moment" and exploring the "world within" caught my eye. I had been practicing sitting meditation for a year or so and had discovered the power of using my breath to stay present, non-judgmentally, without trying to "get somewhere." So even though I felt initially hesitant about T'ai Chi, having always avoided activities which required multiple tasks simultaneously, the idea of carrying over what I'd learned into another type of meditation that involved movement and exercise seemed intriguing. I was initially concerned about coordinating the different parts of my body, enough so that I felt a little out of place at first. But I told myself that at least the moves would be done slowly. Now after six months of practicing the form I can get through the first section on my own, and I'm starting to feel more confident.

Only twice so far, have I felt that wave of energy from the earth traveling up through my body. Even though that feeling eludes me most of the time, there is something about just having felt it that compels me to keep practicing. T'ai Chi calms me down and makes me feel strong, even though part of me remains frustrated at having not yet memorized all the moves. I've also become more comfortable asking for what I need, like additional repetition, or extra practice time after class, in order to learn my moves. I've noticed that the healthier and calmer I feel the more I practice, with the importance I had placed on "being good" having faded somewhat. Outside of class, my concentration has improved, especially in my ability to comprehend what I read without getting distracted. Still, it seems foreign to me to relax muscles, rather than tense them, in order to exert force. And I don't understand what it is about my foot (or whole body) placement that makes my shoes squeak so loudly when attempting to turn in the second section of the form. But I'm beginning to believe Sifu when he says, "Part of the process is learning how to learn. You'll get it eventually." I hope I stick with T'ai Chi. The fact that my experience has been both encouraging and challenging motivates me to continue. I know there will always be something to improve.

Author's notes: This individual begins by talking about unfinished business, which is a common theme in many people's lives as they get older. We often get side tracked from our ideal aspirations by life's harsher realities. In her case this is exacerbated by a mild learning disability. However, she knows how to learn, and T'ai Chi seems somehow to hold a key for her to that which was unfinished. Her account would seem to indicate that she is in the early stages of discovering T'ai Chi's potential role and value toward resolution of her own unfinished business.

Male, age 27. Looking back over the past three years, I'm aware that my view of T'ai Chi has changed dramatically. I had been doing Kung Fu for approximately six years prior to my involvement in T'ai Chi. I only began T'ai Chi because my Sifu stipulated it as a requirement in order to fulfill my ambition to someday become a Kung Fu Sifu with a school of my own. To be honest, I really disliked T'ai Chi at first. I was a Kung Fu teaching assistant and accustomed to hard and fast moves, lots of sweat, and a workout that gave me a cardiovascular rush. I obviously wasn't going to get this from T'ai Chi.

For the first year or so, even though I didn't care for it, I stuck it out with T'ai Chi and continued to show up for class. But that's as far as my enthusiasm went. I suppose I went through what all the other beginners were going through, in that my main concern was just "getting" the moves. With six years of Kung Fu under my belt, remembering the movements to the form wasn't too difficult. It was like any other form I was learning, I would show up, watch my Sifu go through the form, and mirror him to the best of my ability. At that point, I didn't care about any internal feeling, but all that changed when I encountered my teacher's teacher in a weekend seminar intensive.

I don't even recall what the seminar was about, but what I took away from it was a whole new sense of "center" and the feeling that went along with it. Subsequent to that experience, I found that this new feeling of center, along with the many principles that my teacher regularly discussed in class, could actually be interwoven into my Kung Fu practice. Now when I went to my T'ai Chi classes, I found that I was listening as well as watching. Even though I was still trying to remember the form, now I was beginning to attempt to grasp the feelings of inner connection and Ch'i that went along with it.

I can honestly say now, after practicing T'ai Chi for three years, that I have developed a profound respect for it. When I attend classes, I still see myself working to improve my form, but my attention is oriented more to an internal level than it was before. As an external martial artist, my Kung Fu wouldn't be where it is today if I hadn't stuck it out with the T'ai Chi. That goes for the rest of my life as well. Granted, my body and overall physical being have gotten stronger due to T'ai Chi, but my emotions and thought processes have opened up or been awakened also through T'ai Chi. I feel better able to handle my own day to day problems as well as the problems of others.

I believe that as a martial art, T'ai Chi has tools that everyone can benefit from, not just for doing T'ai Chi, but for living life. Through a combination of learning the moves, cultivating my energies, and grasping the theory and principles behind T'ai Chi, I've become more aware of life around me and have gained respect for life (all life) by realizing or seeing how all things affect each other. Based on this, I believe T'ai Chi is the perfect adjunct, for those who practice other martial arts, to add to their practice.

So for me, T'ai Chi has been a life experience that has broadened my horizons and helped me to see things with more respect and understanding. I feel that T'ai Chi is something I will be practicing for as long as I am able.

Author's notes: This personal account speaks eloquently to the issue of T'ai Chi as a companion practice for those involved in harder style martial arts, both from a physical/technical and from a psycho-spiritual perspective. Were it not for the influence of T'ai Chi, this individual would likely still be swimming on the surface, rather than exploring the depths, of his own personal/martial development.

Male, age 60. Let me begin by saying that I've been very sick now with heart problems for four or five years. The upshot was that I wasn't getting much blood to the brain and so my memory loss was quite significant. Along with that my ability to engage in physical activities became more and more limited as time went on. A friend suggested that I take up T'ai Chi. So I read some books on Asian philosophy and the whole idea sounded very interesting. I decided to give it a whirl, but I really wasn't very committed for my first few months of practice. Then I became very ill and went into the hospital for some major operations. At that point, while I was in the hospital lying in bed trying to recover, I remembered I could do my T'ai Chi breathing exercises. The nurse noticed and asked me what I was doing and I said I was doing breathing exercises and that I wanted to get up and try walking in the corridors. From that point I noticed I began regaining my mobility relatively quickly. The next three or four weeks of recovery were actually quite miserable, but I kept getting up and doing what basic T'ai Chi I could remember. I knew I was feeling results and my nurse confirmed that I was way ahead of schedule in my recovery. Well, within six weeks I was back in T'ai Chi class.

This time around my experience of T'ai Chi was quite different. It hit me in an entirely different way. Sifu would point out little things. He would tuck my chin here, straighten my spine, or tap my shoulder to make me relax. I began to become far more aware of my body and realized I was carrying horrible tension. But if I followed his directions I was able to dissipate this tension. This was very wonderful and I began to apply this to my daily life. If I were working on a project I would stop and assess myself and realize there was tension in my shoulder, or that my legs were tight, and I'd stop and relax and do some meditation exercise and just some basic T'ai Chi practice. I found that would change the way I felt entirely and I would get my energy back.

Meanwhile, I kept attending class as often as possible and learning more of the form. I was able to remember the moves much better and it began to snowball. I felt as if was making rapid strides in terms of my overall well-being. Now, I've turned into a real T'ai Chi enthusiast. I'm walking every day and working at my job as a blacksmith, which requires lifting heavy weights, and still attending class four or five times a week, all this just six months after a triple bypass. So I feel that I have definitely gained a lot from T'ai Chi in terms of my attitude, my approach to life, and my ability to relax. I'm also thinking in a more rational manner. T'ai Chi has given me more focus so I'm able to do a lot of the things I hadn't been able to do for ten years or so. I'm extremely pleased.

Another little thing that I find interesting is that I hit a low point, as many of us do, at three or four in the afternoon. I start to slide emotionally, and physically I'm just tired. A snack doesn't help and a nap just puts me in a worse frame of mind. When that happens I stop and I do my T'ai Chi and within an hour my energy is back and I can feel the Ch'i energy coming into my body. It's just flowing through my arms and hands and feet. I've gotten to the point where I can see it in my mind. I can see it as energy moving through my body, a yellow energy that follows me and changes shape, and I can feel its warmth. It's just fascinating. So T'ai Chi has become very special for me. I think people who want to accept the challenge to help themselves along, and to rejuvenate themselves, should really take a good look at it and give it a try.

Author's notes: This account evidences initially, T'ai Chi's propriety as an adjunctive therapeutic modality for those in weakened or recuperative states. It also shows that T'ai Chi breathing and mindfulness skills can be gainfully employed outside of form practice according to special circumstances. This account would also seem to suggest that T'ai Chi can be used to balance mood swings, hormonal variations, and energy levels in a more generalized sense.

Female, age 38. I originally got started at T'ai Chi because I was an oriental bodyworker. Some of my teachers recommended that I get involved with T'ai Chi or Ch'i Kung as a way to enhance the energy flow in my own body. I certainly felt I needed that at that point in my life because none of the disciplines I was involved with for myself were of the body, except for tennis. Even with my tennis I felt I needed to be more grounded. Actually, one of my regular tennis opponents who wasn't that great a player kept beating me. He was just so athletic, which he attributed to his practice of T'ai Chi. He thought T'ai Chi might help my tennis game.

Now I've been practicing T'ai Chi for about two years and I notice a big improvement in my ability to focus, which I definitely credit to T'ai Chi. I especially notice this at tennis where the female opponents I play against in my league are more easily distracted, just like I used to be. But this sense of focusing is something that I notice elsewhere in my life as well as on the tennis court.

As a professional bodyworker I'm pretty sensitive to where I hold blocks and tensions in my own body. T'ai Chi seems somehow to amplify those, or at least my awareness of them. I feel chronic tension in my shoulder, for example, which I notice when I'm practicing. It's frustrating at times that I still have some of these issues after so many years of doing my own work. But now at least I know where I hold my tension. I'm also pretty sensitive on an emotional level, knowing that I've had anger issues to be resolved. Sometimes T'ai Chi can bring that stuff right up to the surface for me where it can linger unresolved. So this can feel pretty challenging at times, working through all this stuff. The good thing is that I'm more self-aware so that I can keep breathing and just stay with my own process. I figure that at least it's coming up to where I can work with it, which is a lot better than the alternative of its staying repressed in my body, perhaps to manifest at some later time as illness.

I've trained at quite a range of healing modalities, including yoga, hypnotherapy, reiki, astrology, and acupressure, besides having a degree in counseling psychology. I feel that T'ai Chi is particularly empowering because it's something you can learn to do for yourself without needing to have it done to you or for you by another practitioner. After I've had a good session at T'ai Chi class I feel as if I've been through a bodywork treatment. I've found that T'ai Chi is a good way to run energy through my body.

I'm continually impressed at the quality of my own energy experiences with T'ai Chi, particularly given my own earlier experiences as a reiki practitioner. I'd say there's no comparison. I feel ten times the energy with T'ai Chi and Ch'i Kung than I felt through the practice of my earlier disciplines. I really like that feeling of Ch'i running through my meridians, through my palms, and being able to ground and root to the earth and pull the earth's energy up. For me, that sensory experience of moving energy through my body is a high point of my practice.

Author's notes: Again, as in one of the earlier accounts, the point is made that health care providers, regardless of whether their practice is conventional or alternative, need to attend to themselves in order to be of reliable service to others. T'ai Chi can be of inestimable value in this regard. The application of T'ai Chi's principles to other activities, such as tennis or golf remains, for the most part, unexplored but in my mind, begs further attention.

CONCLUSION

As I read over the personal accounts above, which were submitted by my students, I personally am impressed by the diverse spectrum of feelings and experiences they have shared as to how their lives have been affected by their practice of T'ai Chi. But what impressed me even more, caught me a bit off guard actually, was how much of what they shared was new information to me, that with all my emphasis on "process" there remained so much hidden from view even in regards to my own students. I think therein lies a lesson for us teachers, that our students are students only second, first they are unique and multi-faceted individuals who should never be taken for granted.

CHAPTER 15

Lectures and Musings

This chapter is comprised of transcripts of selected class lectures, focusing on various large or small aspects of the T'ai Chi experience, that I have delivered to my own students over the years. Mixed in with the lecture transcripts (more or less verbatim, except for informational clarity adjustments) are some personal musings apropos to the topic. You will likely notice that some of the material covered here is also addressed elsewhere in this book. I don't mind repeating myself some as it is often the case that varying the delivery even slightly, of otherwise same or similar information can have a profound effect on how it is heard or received by the student. I know for myself that hearing a new descriptive phrase, analogy, or metaphor can expand the way I perceive knowledge or information already held deeply within.

You may also notice that some of what follows borders, how shall I say, on the fringes of T'ai Chi, which is exactly why it's here in "Lectures and Musings" rather than elsewhere in this book. Sometimes T'ai Chi is just about T'ai Chi, and sometimes T'ai Chi is about everything.

HEALTHY FEET/HAPPY FEET

Our feet provide the very foundation for our T'ai Chi, connecting us down to the Earth, allowing us to root throughout our practice, and in fact, throughout our lives. Yet despite this important role, the feet are seldom paid any special heed beyond attention to their correct placement and positioning during form practice. Indeed, the feet are usually quite taken for granted.

Every now and then during class, I like to sit my students down and have everyone remove their shoes and socks in order to pay close attention to the state of their feet. We use this opportunity to massage the feet, your own or somebody else's, using reflexology techniques to explore for and attend to any painful trigger points or crystalline lactic acid deposits. We can also use this opportunity to practice techniques (which I'll explain shortly) for strengthening the feet and improving small muscle coordination. Fifteen or twenty minutes of this every now and then is time well spent and never fails to leave students amazed at the results once they stand up to resume their form practice.

It is very common for stress and tension to accumulate in the feet. Take a minute to reflect and you will agree that the feet are probably the most used and abused parts of our bodies. Many people are on their feet all day long, often on unyielding floor or ground surfaces. This is a far cry from times of yore when people walked barefoot or lightly shod across the earth's surface. Today, hard floors, repetitive tasks, and ill-fitting or over worn shoes, greatly exacerbate the stress and tension that get stored in our feet.

In my mind this comprises a compelling argument for good footwear as a means to good health in general. This is particularly the case for activities such as T'ai Chi where healthy, happy feet are so important to the overall quality of your practice. Barring any opportunity to work barefoot on the earth, I always encourage my students to wear lightweight flat-soled shoes that afford them support in all directions. Cross training type shoes are often suitable to this task. Also, there are several martial arts shoes currently on the market that meet these criteria nicely. The fact that designers are fickle and often withdraw perfectly good shoes from the market in favor of next generation designs, is a problem which precludes my endorsing any particular shoe here. A type of shoe which I specifically do not recommend however, is the traditional slipper type Kung Fu/T'ai Chi shoes. Although they can be worn comfortably by some people, these slippers offer little traction and no support. Anybody wearing them who has any predisposition to foot, knee, or back problems will likely find those problems eventually aggravated by their footwear.

One of the best ways to insure healthy happy feet is to implement the following exercises occasionally into your warm-up routine. At first these exercises may require a chunk of your time, but once you know them five minutes is all the time you will need.

#1 **Toe Pick Ups.** Find yourself five small objects (marbles, small corks, pistachio nuts, etc.) and place them on the floor near and to the inside of one of your feet. Sit or stand and begin with any toe. Pick up and grasp one object with one toe and hold it while you pivot on the heel to turn your foot outward. Then ease your grip to release the object down. Repeat this procedure with each of your other toes until all the objects have been moved out to the side. Then, reverse the process, using your toes to return the objects to their starting positions. If your toes aren't too tired yet, and you're not too frustrated, start over. Once your toes get tired switch to your other foot and repeat. At first, this task may seem nearly impossible, but in just a few practice sessions you should improve your fine muscle control considerably and, at the very least, be able to impress your friends at parties.

#2 **Scrunching.** Place a towel flat on the floor and stand barefoot at its edge. Now use your toes to scrunch the towel, gathering it up under your feet. If no towel is handy stand barefoot on a carpeted surface and use your toes (no cheating with body rocking) to pull yourself across the floor.

#3 **Heel Lifts (with or without shoes).**
    a) Stand straight with your feet flat and toes forward. Lift up off your heels on to your toes. Repeat in sets of ten.

    b) Flare your feet and toes well outward (heels in) and repeat the same lifting pattern.

    c) Finally turn the feet/toes/knees inward (heels out) and repeat in the same manner.

#4 Foot Rolling—Stand straight with your feet flat, toes forward, and roll each foot to the outside onto the "blade" edge of the foot. Repeat a set or sets before reversing to roll the foot in. Note: You will probably notice a greater degree of flexibility when rolling the feet out as compared to rolling them in.

These exercises will have the effect of both stretching and strengthening the small muscles and other soft tissues of the feet. Combine these with the reflexology foot massage (any book on reflexology can familiarize you with its details if you really get into it) and you will find an enhanced sensitivity of your feet allowing for greater enjoyment of the T'ai Chi form and improved rooting abilities.

T'AI CHI STANDING

The simplest and most basic stance in T'ai Chi involves standing upright, as is the case with the beginning and closing positions at either end of the T'ai Chi form. Yet even with something as simple as "just standing" there are misconceptions about how to do it right, that is to say in accordance with T'ai Chi principles. I once had a fellow who had been practicing T'ai Chi for over fifteen years participate in a workshop I was conducting. The man had horrible posture, but the shame of it was that he had striven consciously to develop his posture based on his (mis)interpretation of the advice given in the T'ai Chi Classics. He had sunk his shoulders and raised his back to the point that he looked almost like a hunchback, and nothing that I could say seemed to have any effect on his way of thinking. By the time I came along he was thoroughly invested in his posture and had neither the desire to change nor any inclination to consider why he should.

The advice given in the Classics can be easily misinterpreted by those who aren't sufficiently experienced at T'ai Chi to discern the subtler meanings. For example, the Classics also advise us to sink our Ch'i in order to remain rooted to the earth, and to simultaneously raise the *Bai Hui* point so as to open and extend the spine. This advice can be (reasonably) misconstrued to mean that we should stand up perfectly straight. However, standing perfectly straight neither opens the spine nor reinforces our connection to the earth. The following illustration (see Figure 15-1, left side) depicts how standing up too straight allows for an efficient transfer of energy only from top to bottom or vice versa. Structuring yourself like this is of limited value in T'ai Chi. By standing up too straight you deny yourself the opportunity for an optimally efficient transfer of incoming force down through your body to the earth. Force coming in from any other direction than directly overhead will carry you along with it as it passes through your body.

The more correct way to stand entails a slight opening (separation) of the shoulder blades that will naturally roll both the shoulders and the upper thoracic

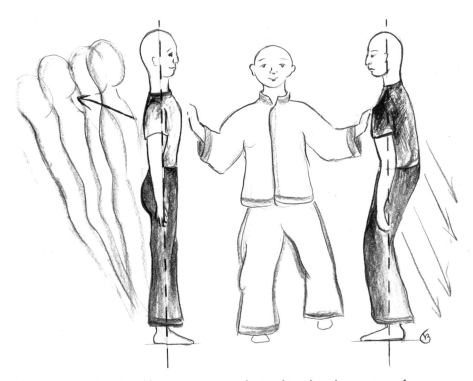

Figure 15-1 (left side). Holding your stance overly straight and rigid prevents you from connecting firmly to the earth. **Figure 15-2 (right side).** Settling your stance allows you to stay better rooted to the earth and allows for more versatility in adjusting to incoming forces.

vertebrae slightly forward. The chest will hollow automatically like a sail on a sailboat catching a gentle breeze and the spine will arch just ever-so-slightly to lengthen from tailbone to *Bai Hui*. The illustration (see Figure 15-2, right side) shows how a wider range of incoming forces from either the front or back can thus be more efficiently transferred down through the body to the earth.

It is important to remember as well that your technical articulation can be enhanced by being deliberately attentive to feeling/imagining a connection between the Bubbling Well points of your feet and your perineum and also between your tailbone and your *Bai Hui* point. Paying attention to these connections will help to nudge your experience of standing from the realm of body balance only into the higher realm of energy work.

HOW A WORM DRIVES

Let's take a closer look at the move Ward Off. The body mechanics of this move are fascinating. Thinking about this move brings to mind for me a time when I was a lot younger, in my post-hippie days, when as a young(er) idealist I lived on a small farm in New England. It wasn't a working farm per se but I gardened food crops with great enthusiasm, to the point that one year I went out and purchased a Troy-Bilt Roto-Tiller. I chose the Troy-Bilt over other brands because I was convinced it was the best quality Roto-Tiller on the market. While some tillers were chain driven (like a bicycle) and others were sprocket-gear or belt driven, the Troy-Bilt alone used a worm drive to transfer power from its engine to the earth breaking tines in front. It's the concept of a worm drive that calls to my mind the T'ai Chi move, Ward Off.

A worm gear itself is a straight or conical shaft with either recessed grooves or external ridges that are spiraled (not unlike a common hardware screw.) The rotation of these grooves or ridges affords an optimally efficient transfer of power. The fact that this type of gear is very durable as well, makes it the preferred choice for applications that require impelling force through any anticipated resistance. Thus, besides its application in the Troy-Bilt Roto-Tiller, the worm drive is commonly found in electric drills, propeller drive shafts and, as mentioned earlier, in the form of common hardware screws. Perhaps the most impressive testimony to their mechanical superiority is the use of worm drives in the equipment used for drilling roadway tunnels through the earth.

If you've ever actually used a Roto-Tiller to turn fresh ground you know you're bound to hit some resistance, rocks or clumps of clay, or tightly bound sod. If the Roto-Tines are struggling against the earth, their thwarted power has got to go somewhere, and that somewhere is most logically back through the machine towards the source of power. Whatever is the weakest link in the system will thus be under great stress. Chains, sprocket gears or belts can bend, break, slip, or simply wear out under constant strain. No problem with a worm drive. It's a solid unit, just turn it and it drives.

The same can be said for Ward Off. In the Ward Off move your feet and legs are like an engine, generating power to be expressed as force spiraling up through the body and outward. The degree of spiraling may vary according to how different people practice their form. However that spiraling force is always there, so that everything between your feet and that point where force leaves your body can be likened to the screw-like spiraling force of a worm drive.

There is however an important consideration that cannot be overlooked. You must be careful to keep your body properly aligned at all times lest your force go awry. If you've ever tried screw a hardware screw that was bent even just slightly out of shape into a piece of wood, you know it's nearly impossible to direct your drive force efficiently through the screw. The same can said for Ward Off. In order for the technique to work according to its design, the body must be held properly aligned from the source of force at the earth all the way through to completion.

THE EYES HAVE IT

There are divergent views, if you will, on just exactly what is the role that the eyes play in T'ai Chi, and how that role is fulfilled. Most obviously, we think of the eyes as utile to the extent that they provide us with information about the world outside of and around us. This information is very important from a martial perspective and also for practical living in general.

While practicing T'ai Chi your eyes should be soft yet alert, attuned both to what is before them and sensitive as well to peripheral data. As soft as the eyes should be during T'ai Chi practice it is still important that you develop the ability to convey out through your eyes the unmistakable determination of martial spirit, that quality known as *Yi*, instantly and on demand according to circumstances as they may arise. The better T'ai Chi practitioners with whom I am personally familiar are all able to switch on a "Look", the likes of which will make any opponent think twice. So far, the information I've shared with you can be said to describe the *external* role of the eyes.

It is my experience that the eyes also have an *internal* role that can manifest as a complement to their external role. Your eyes, or perhaps more accurately your mind's eye, can be instrumental in perceiving that which is within. It may seem a little contrived or awkward at first, but you can learn to use your mind's eye to observe experiences or states of being within your body or your mind that would normally be relegated to the visual realm rather than to kinesthetic or cognitive perception. For those of you who are experienced at meditation this shouldn't come as news.

I know that what has been very helpful for me is to visually scan different parts of my body during practice, checking to see if my joints are open, watching my breath, and simply observing myself as if I were on the outside looking in. In practicing to develop this skill it will probably be easier at first if you close your eyes, but eventually as you hone your perceptive abilities you will find that external and internal visual awarenesses are not mutually incompatible.

HOW WE LEARN BY OSMOSIS

Osmosis is the term I use to describe that subtle process of absorption that occurs almost inadvertently by virtue of practicing in the presence of your teacher and fellow classmates. It is learning that occurs somehow adjunct to any conscious and deliberate attempt to take in new information.

When you are involved in a study of T'ai Chi, learning actually occurs on many levels simultaneously. This is important to recognize because T'ai Chi is different from many other kinds of learning as it involves a non-linear learning process. With many other learning approaches, such as cognitive or physical skill development, you typically proceed in your learning in a step-by-step fashion. But with T'ai Chi the learnings register on different tiers throughout your body/mind, often below the level of conscious awareness. One possible downside to this is that those people who are oriented solely towards a goal of measurable or tangible progress will be less likely to recognize and appreciate their "process" for all that it is. These people will be more likely to experience frustration in their attempts to learn. So it's helpful to keep an open mind and an open agenda.

In my own teaching I usually have the entire class, even those who may be brand new at T'ai Chi, follow along as I lead through the first section of the form, or perhaps even the form in its entirety. Reasonably, those students who are newer cannot be expected to recall all or perhaps even any of the movements covered. Does this mean you haven't learned anything in that lesson? Certainly not, though it may feel that way at the time. Well below the level of your conscious awareness the movements that you have practiced are starting to take hold so that with each successive round of practice those movements will both become and feel less unfamiliar. With continued practice the movements of the form will start to coalesce into a familiar whole.

Much of what you are learning here is processed in ways other than by cognitive absorption. Your body has its own intelligence. Over the years, I have been involved with different learning formats, either with teachers in this field per se or in academia. During lectures I always took notes of what was being said or displayed, but 99% of the time I never gave those notes a second look after writing them down. At first glance it seemed a waste to take notes that were destined to be ignored but somehow, jotting them down was helpful. Eventually I came to realize that it was the taking of notes, the actual physical process of committing them to paper, that allowed me to register kinesthetically the information I was receiving audibly or visually.

So it is with T'ai Chi. You may think you're just learning the movements comprising an age-old Chinese exercise system, but T'ai Chi has the potential to affect you at every level of your being.

T'AI CHI FOR KIDS?

I frequently field inquiries from parents anxious to get their kids, sometimes as young as four or five years of age, involved in T'ai Chi, usually for its reputed calming and focusing benefits. Though I'm not unilaterally opposed to T'ai Chi for children I generally dissuade parents from this course of action, recommending that they opt instead for martial activities that are more "out there" in terms of their cerebral orientation, activities such as Kung Fu or Karate. It is true that the kids with whom I've shared T'ai Chi have just loved it. But, in almost all cases the context of that sharing has been some sort of introductory presentation through the schools or community action groups. Kids always love novelty. So, as long as T'ai Chi is novel it will hold the attention of those children who practice it. However, once the novelty wears off and it becomes evident that T'ai Chi is a discipline requiring time, effort and commitment, interest in T'ai Chi may wane in favor of activities offering more immediate gratification. Nor do I regard this as altogether unhealthy; the nature of childhood is, after all, to discover the world around. There's plenty of time for the rigors of introspective discipline once the external world has been given a once over.

In all fairness to parents, I generally applaud their interest in T'ai Chi for their kids. These parents usually have their hearts in the right place. With learning disabilities and ADHD endemic among today's youth parents are well motivated to search out more natural and less invasive treatment modalities as alternatives to the prevailing trend of psycho-pharmacological treatment, which is usually palliative at best. I do favor natural alternatives to chemical intervention whenever and wherever appropriate, but in most cases, at least in the context of an adult class atmosphere, T'ai Chi represents too cerebral a discipline for children. Perhaps if there were a T'ai Chi class just for kids, their developmental idiosyncrasies could be adequately catered to. Hmmm, now there's an idea to be considered. That said though, I feel the mid-teenage years are usually a good minimum age to embark on a study of T'ai Chi in an adult class environment.

THE SEEMING DOWNSIDE OF NEW INFORMATION—ONE STEP BACK FOR TWO FORWARD

It is quite common for T'ai Chi students to find themselves frustrated by their own learning process at various points early on in their training. Despite the inherent slowness of T'ai Chi it sometimes seems to students as if they're being bowled over by an onslaught of new information. The reason for this is because T'ai Chi can represent such a dramatic contrast to, and departure from, information already held. The fact that everything is so inter-connected in T'ai Chi means that once you've got it down right, it's very right, but until you do have it right flaws in your practice can seem to have a systemic impact on your skill overall.

Frustration can occur particularly when you're going along with your practice, just feeling as if you are finally starting to get a more solid grasp of your lessons and your teacher comes along and says, "No, this needs to be done differently." In that moment it can seem as if everything you have learned up to that point falls apart while you pay attention to the new correction. It almost feels as if you are taking a step backwards because everything in T'ai Chi is so interwoven that, when one component is shown to be flawed, it calls everything else into question. In addition, the amount of attention devoted to the new lesson or correction, may be such that it appears to detract from your practice experience overall.

I can relate because this has certainly been my own experience over years past. I can recall how I would think I had something pretty good only to have my teacher say, "No, that's wrong, you've got to change that," and bang, it felt as if I was starting all over again from square one. Certainly there were times when I felt quite discouraged with my practice. Fortunately my feelings of discouragement were usually short lived and tended to dissipate once I remembered to keep my ego in check. In this sense, a step back may be illusory, but sometimes, even backwards is forwards.

The Power of a Smile

A simple smile is perhaps the most underrated variable in the scheme of your T'ai Chi Ch'uan experience and, by extension, in your life. This is because a smile can both reflect and influence the true essence of your practice. Just as your eyes are able to convey outward the power of your intention, whether it be warm regard or the *Yi* of your warrior spirit, so can a smile effectively disarm the walls and defenses of those who would (in some cases reasonably) guard against you, including yourself.

Certainly a smile is more than just an expression on your face. Rather, it is the manifestation of a heartfelt contentment, a small celebration of life itself, and as such, it has a place in T'ai Chi. A true smile, though it may be blatant for all to see, or at times more subtle, requires no overt declaration. A T'ai Chi smile is like that of the Mona Lisa, implying an inward state of acceptance and grace, and a place of balance in the Tao.

During my practice there are times when I just notice I am smiling, sometimes to the point that I have to contain myself (as when I'm teaching and feel that a smile might distract or miscue my students). Other times I notice that I am not smiling when I really ought to be, and this realization can help me to become more aware of stress or tension being held in my body/mind that needs to be addressed.

We usually think of a smile as reflecting what is already there, perhaps some inner state, but you can actually cultivate your own smile as a way of inducing its alchemical effects to influence, rather than merely reflect, what it is that's going on inside. A smile is one way of triggering your body/mind's relaxation response as a component of the parasympathetic nervous system. This can be done anytime, not just during T'ai Chi practice. But if you make it a point to explore the potential of your smile during your form practice you may well discover a new practice tool at your disposal.

Surface Tension

New T'ai Chi students are often frustrated at the apparent paradox of softness within hardness and vice versa. It's usually not the concept of softness being able to overcome hardness that is difficult to grasp. Most people actually find the concept quite romantic in that it seems to conjure up the very ideals of Eastern philosophy. It is the practical integration of that concept into one's practice that seems to stymie less experienced practitioners. So many of us are invested in the belief and the experience that effort produces results, and that more effort produces more or better results. In most cases this both stems from, and is reinforced by, the experiences we've had in our lives, academically, vocationally, and particularly in sports.

As is often the case with Eastern disciplines, our natural environment lends itself to analogies or metaphors that can be invoked to catalyze our practical grasp of difficult concepts. The idea is that naturally occurring models can inspire a shift in our own practice paradigm. If something happens in nature it must not be impossible.

In nature we have the water droplet, which manifests a sufficiently consistent shape and form that it is its own description. Why are droplets "droplets", and not random splatters? Water is usually regarded as a paragon of softness, as the most yielding element. Yet it still has enough strength to hold itself together in what science recognizes to be an extraordinarily efficient and minimally energy intensive form. The answer has to do with surface tension. As soft as water is, its surface tension is such that a needle placed on its (flat) surface will float as easily as would a cork or a boat.

Chemistry offers its own explanation for this phenomenon as distinct from T'ai Chi. Nevertheless I find it helpful, in striving for softness within, to liken my own external self to the surface tension of water. I think of having just enough, no more and no less, outside tension to hold together that which is within. In this manner I am able to feel a power contained within, soft in its latency, yet explosive in its potential.

BOX OF CHOCOLATES, OR SLICE OF PIE

Students often ask me if T'ai Chi can really make a difference in their lives. They want to know if it can help them to become better people? If so, how so, and how much so? In order to shed a clearer light on T'ai Chi's potential to serve us in this manner, I liken life to pie, a whole pie with an infinite number of possible slices. Each individual slice represents the realization potential, for better or worse, of any given person. Some slices in the pie might be bigger, smaller, or further away, and more clearly separate from the slices of particular others. Some pie slices may overlap, even to the point of nearly merging. But, no two slices are exactly alike because each of us is unique in who we are, and in who we can become. Contained within each of our slices is the sum total, not only of who we are, but who we have been, and who we might become.

As you think of these pie slices, let yourself imagine that the left side of each slice represents the absolute God-like best that we could possibly become in this life. Let the right side represent the unspeakable worst manifestation of our human potential. Most people wallow somewhere in the middle, perhaps a bit more to one side or the other of center. T'ai Chi as a self realization tool for body and soul, can help us to move further and further to the left of center so that we are continually improving ourselves, always becoming better and better, towards a realization of our fullest and best human potential. No one of us can ever be the same as anyone else but, within the framework of our own pie slice, we can optimize our existence. "Better and better," of course is a relative concept, including both quantitative and qualitative features. Examples of quantitative features include posture and carriage, the absence of blatant pathology, and, regarding T'ai Chi, an accomplishment and embodiment of standards and principles commonly associated with mastery of the practice. Qualitative features include a sense of personal fulfillment, emotional balance, and some resolution as regards your own greater purpose in life. I answer with a resounding, "Yes!" T'ai Chi can indeed make a difference in the lives of those who embrace its practice. T'ai Chi can help you to become independently healthy.

T'AI CHI AS A HEALING ART

For many years now I've been a proponent of T'ai Chi as a healing art. Of course the T'ai Chi literature is rife with stories of this master or that master who, after a sickly childhood or being diagnosed with some debilitating condition, undertook a study of T'ai Chi only to enjoy renewed health and longevity. Such accounts, though largely empirical, are certainly inspiring. I have juxtaposed accounts such as these with my own direct experience of energy healing methods employed by various teachers I have worked with, always looking for those threads common to the many different approaches that have been developed over time. Some teachers/healers rely on patting/palpation. Others employ shaking methods, and I've heard several variations of martial/healing sounds. Then of course, there is acupuncture, moxabustion, et al., two methods with which most people are at least peripherally familiar.

What each of these different approaches to healing seems to have in common is a presumptive reliance on vibration, or frequency, or wavelength. Whether it's the heat of moxabustion, the slow movement of tissue through palpation, or the vibration of sound, on some level a frequency is established to (at)tune the organism. I don't know a great deal about physics but I find this idea fascinating because it seems to me as if this is somehow at the core of everything, not just Eastern healing arts, but everything. Even Western medicine and technology appear to be coming full circle in recognition that frequency represents a new frontier with infinite potential. Heat, movement, light, and sound are all different expressions of the same thing. Now as I said, I'm not a physicist, so I don't want to get out of my depth, but it seems to me that T'ai Chi, by virtue of its emphasis on balancing and cultivating your Ch'i and of being in harmony with yourself, and by extension with your environment, and by further extension with the Tao, is one way of coming more into alignment with powerful universal forces (frequencies) in ways that are both existential and quite practical.

Musicians know that by sounding a single keynote on a piano, the same keynote on other pianos in close proximity will sound spontaneously. This is known as morphic resonance. Similarly, it is known in Classical Homeopathy, a non-allopathic medical modality, that certain toxic substances can be prepared (diluted and vibrationally potentized) to efficaciously treat the very same or similar symptoms that they would normally induce in their more naturally occurring states. Thus it seems reasonable to me that the subtle energetic vibrations that we create as a result of correct T'ai Chi practice, whether from the actual physical movements or from the energy of clear and healthy intentions, have the potential to align us harmonically with the Tao, and so restore and/or maintain our body/minds as optimally functioning entities.

T'AI CHI AND OLD BONES

Traditionally T'ai Chi has been regarded as an appropriate form of exercise for the elderly. Aside from the fact that T'ai Chi is slow and non-jarring, there are two less obvious reasons as to why T'ai Chi can be of particular benefit to older people. Both these reasons entail a very direct impact on the bones of those who practice. Bone health is a very real issue for those past middle age. Statistics show that approximately 15% of men and 30% of all women suffer from hip fracture before age ninety.[1] Even discounting hip fractures, injuries having to do with bones are simply pandemic in our society, and on the rise. This is due both to age related declines in balance and equilibrium, and also to bones that have become weakened through bone loss.

In the first case, empirical evidence has long indicated what clinical research has now proven conclusively, that T'ai Chi is one the best, if not the best, methods for improving balance in the elderly thus preventing falls.[2]

Second, it is common knowledge that older people are at great risk for bone loss. Women in particular, are at risk by a factor of two to four times compared to men for loss in bone density. Post-menopausal women can lose bone mass at up to 1% per year. However this is not just a woman's issue. Male astronauts stationed in space for extended periods have been found to lose bone density at a rate of 1% per month! Now you may not be an astronaut, but the point is that this accelerated bone loss in astronauts occurs simply by virtue of their not being exposed to the natural stress of gravity here on earth. One study showed that patients confined to bed rest following back injury, can lose lumbar bone mass at up to 1% per week.[3] This suggests that bone mass (growth or loss) is to a very great degree stress dependent, and that bone growth/density can actually be encouraged, or at least maintained, via healthy stressors.

Current research indicates that osteoporotic bone loss is a lifestyle disease stemming from a range of factors, including diet and exercise. Ironically it is much more prevalent in prosperous first world countries than in less technologically advanced societies. Healthy exercise has been shown conclusively to be a key to healthy bones. In fact lack of proper exercise actually reduces the ability of bones to self-repair.[4]

T'ai Chi practice can strengthen bones directly. Because of its emphasis on exact and efficient skeletal alignment, T'ai Chi takes the stress of gravity off the muscles and puts it back where it belongs...on the bones. So elderly practitioners of T'ai Chi get to double dip, so to speak. The cumulative effects of regular and correct T'ai Chi practice over time will improve their balance on the one hand, and strengthen their bones at the same time.

BOUNCE BACK FORCE

An important consideration in learning how to use your T'ai Chi for pushing or for practical self-defense, is *bounce back force,* or echo force. Any time you issue force outward there is always some level of resistance encountered. Unless you happen to be in a vacuum, there will always be resistance. Even when you're practicing without an actual physical target there is resistance from the air, though it's hardly perceptible because the resistance is slight and we're accustomed to it.

When you press or push into a real somebody or something the resistance is more pronounced. In much the same way that sonar or radar waves bounce back from any object encountered, your force, when issued out, means a certain amount of echo force will bounce back in. There are two reasons why this bounce back force is an important consideration. First, bounce back force will naturally lodge, whether or not it is actually felt, at whatever place in your body represents the weakest link. So, if in issuing force your posture is weak, the echo force will lodge back within you causing some degree of structural collapse or strain. This can result in a loss of balance or possibly an injury. Second, bounce back force can mean that your own power fails to be directed efficiently where you intend for it to go, thus rendering your technique versus your opponent less effective.

If your posture and alignment are correct, your body will be more stable and less prone to injury. Any bounce back force will simply reverberate back to your opponent, much like an echo bouncing back and forth between two walls. Thus, you need to develop a sensitivity to the way force travels through your body, as well as to your "follow up", just as you would in tennis or golf, insuring that each technique is executed correctly and to its full completion. In this manner you can avoid being the unintended recipient of your own force. The idea is pretty basic and simple, but getting it is not.

INTELLIGENT T'AI CHI

In addition to T'ai Chi having a direct positive impact on neurological function in terms of how the brain is hardwired, that is to say how the brain *facilitates* intelligence, I don't think it's too much of a stretch to say that T'ai Chi can promote intelligence in more ways then one. Back in 1983 Harvard researcher Howard Gardner proposed an alternative view to the Stanford-Binet IQ test as the standard measurement of individual intelligence. Prior to Gardner's work, intelligence had been ascribed to the exclusive realm of cognitive function. Gardner proposed that there were actually seven discernible forms of intelligence, including body-kinesthetic, spatial, interpersonal, intra-personal, musical, linguistic, and logical-mathematical.[4]

It is my opinion that individual intelligence is determined by both internal and external factors and it can be both innate and cultivated (nature *and* nurture). Certain activities or trainings promote the development of particular types of these various intelligences. For example, participating in sports primarily promotes kinesthetic intelligence, and can also possibly contribute to spatial intelligence, because it is not just one's body that one is concerned with but the performance of that body in a spatial context. This would particularly be so in the case of team sports where there are many fluid variables to be taken into account within a dynamic versus static context.

Another activity might be practicing the piano, which primarily promotes musical intelligence, and to the extent that the fingers are involved, kinesthetic intelligence.

I believe that T'ai Chi very directly facilitates the development of several different types of intelligence. Most obviously T'ai Chi operates in the kinesthetic realm, but also requires spatial orientation in a very deliberate and conscientious, versus instinctive, manner. Many sports favor participants with spatial intelligence but offer little in the way of its deliberate cultivation. T'ai Chi, by virtue of its emphasis on total body attunement, both to the self and to the immediate environment, compels spatial awareness. Further, if T'ai Chi is fully exploited as a spiritual or personal development discipline the insights it can afford are clear evidence of its ability to foster intra-personal intelligence, or knowledge and understanding of the self. Less directly, T'ai Chi can be said to promote interpersonal intelligence (enhanced communication with others, albeit in this case non-verbal) due to its emphasis in Pushing Hands practice both on (receiving) listening to and perceiving the energy and intention of another person and (sending) communicating information judiciously with whomever one might be working.

Let me take this a step further by suggesting that these various intelligences, just like cognitive intelligence, have a use plasticity. The more you use them the more, and more efficiently, you will be able to use them. So if you want to be real smart, do T'ai Chi.

THE YIN AND YANG SIDES OF T'AI CHI, AND T'AI CHI STUDENTS

One of the challenges for students and teachers alike is striking a balance between the two defining features of T'ai Chi, its external and its internal manifestations. On the Yang side we have T'ai Chi from a perspective of technical expertise, a form sequence that ideally looks and feels perfect. On the Yin side we have T'ai Chi as an internal energetic experience, entailing a state of body/mind that aspires to balanced health and to energy pathways that are open and free of obstruction. Though the obvious goal is a process that allows you to acquire an integrated command of both sides of the equation, it has been my experience that neither side is entirely contingent on the other, and that until you reach an advanced level of practice it's quite unlikely that you will be fully balanced in your command of both these aspects.

By virtue of my dual role as Kung Fu Sifu and T'ai Chi teacher I have an opportunity to work with two relative extremes of incoming students, as well as those representing a middle ground. On the one hand, those Kung Fu students of mine who are most talented inevitably develop an interest in T'ai Chi at some point. These are motivated individuals who bring to T'ai Chi a highly developed musculoskeletal expertise in terms of their ability to tell their bodies what to do and then have their bodies respond accordingly. They may however, have little sense of internal dynamics in terms of Ch'i and psyche. On the other hand I seem to attract, as I'm sure do many other T'ai Chi teachers, a disproportionate number of students already oriented towards energy awareness and healing arts such as bodyworkers, psychotherapists, meditators, and energy healers representing various modalities. This population of students often displays a predisposition, at the very least, to mindfulness and energy cultivation, even prior to embarking on any study of T'ai Chi. The challenges that each of these two factions are faced with can be quite different. This can be challenging as well for the teacher whose job it is to address a broad range of needs and abilities in any given class in order to insure that all students get what they need to develop internally and externally.

Not only are those features and pre-dispositions that define these two separate camps not contingent on each other, but either one can hypothetically, be cultivated in the absence, or even to the exclusion, of the other. It would be quite possible during a course of study to emphasize either just the technical aspects of T'ai Chi or its internal energetic qualities. Of course, this is not something you would strive for, but it can be reassuring to know that T'ai Chi need not be an "all or nothing" experience. Nobody should feel that just because they lack a well-developed skill at one aspect of T'ai Chi their practice is for naught.

If you happen to be someone who understands, even feels energy, but your moves are awkward and unbalanced—maybe you just don't seem to be getting it—don't despair. Enjoy what strengths you do have and just keep oriented towards the process of learning the moves correctly. If you're not getting something there are reasons for it, and with continued time and practice (and competent instruction) those reasons will become clearer and you will improve. Sooner or later, once you are ready, you will get what you need.

The same can be said for physically talented individuals lacking an internal orientation. Actually it can be a bit more trying for people who are used to their efforts producing more immediate results. Some aspects of internal development simply cannot be rushed. It's like the old story where the prospective Student asks the Master how long it will take to learn, and the Master replies, "five years". The Student asks, "What if I practice diligently?" to which the Master replies, "ten years." The student then asks, "Suppose I train all day, everyday?" "in that case, just fifteen years," answers the Master.

Sometimes, you just have to able to surrender control in order to get what you want. This is one example of what is called "investing in loss." There is a difference between losing and investing in loss. By definition, an investment entails an expenditure that one hopes will eventually yield positive results. So it is with the practice of T'ai Chi.

NATURAL REFLECTIONS

I have a few things to draw to your attention as we move through just the first section of the form. Let's start from the beginning with the very first move, the T'ai Chi Open Stance, in which you simply raise the hands prior to stepping off. When raising the arms and hands you want to simultaneously press your Bubbling Well points down into the earth. This downward press into your feet will lend a wavelike quality to your body and arms as you raise the arms up in front. You'll feel this wave of force traveling up through your body and out to your fingertips before it returns back down through your body to the earth, (the returning down part being somewhat analogous to an undertow). Though there are no corners per se, the hands and fingertips are where that wavelike force changes direction from "up and out" to "back in and down". In order to really feel this quality you can exaggerate the movement of the hands as the fingers extend out and up so that they resemble the tail fin of a whale propelling itself forward through the ocean's depths.

Next we'll work on Brush Knee and Push, paying particular attention to the Push component. Again you'll feel how force travels from the earth up through your body in a wavelike motion and out the arm to your palm. In the case of this move the wrist hinge is critical. As you lift the "Push" hand up to shoulder height and start to bring it forward, let your fingers lead, pulling the hand and arm along behind, while holding your wrist somewhat in reserve. Complete the Push component by catching your wrist up with its palm in order to concentrate the full force of your blow at the *Lao Kung* point. The mechanics of this move remind me of the principle behind those small notched sticks that primitive man developed to increase the power and distance of a thrown spear. Spear throwers, or atlatls as they were known in the more recent Aztec culture, acted as hinged extensions to their weapons. The snapping action of their hinged release gave primitive man a distinct advantage at combat or hunting. The same principle of a hinged release will add exponentially to the power latent in your pushing hand in the Brush Knee move.

Now let's examine Play the Guitar. In this move we employ a double wave of force. The right side of the body, leading with the right arm, reaches forward, pulls up, and then rolls back, its force returning down through the body to the earth. Simultaneously, the left side wave rolls its force in almost the same way, but the timing is exactly opposite that of the right side. The image that comes to mind for me here is that of the wheels of a train with their drive and coupling-rod assemblies moving in an alternating tandem to drive the train's wheels. Such an image is powerful indeed.

Finally let's look at Twist and Strike. As you twist to bring your right arm up the left side of your body the right elbow is as the crest of a wave force. As you draw your elbow upward it pulls its own fist along behind in tow, with the left palm trailing behind. It's as if the elbow were clearing the way for the right fist, and the right fist in turn clearing the way for the left palm, the left palm content to follow in its wake. The unraveling quality of this move always makes me think of bicycle racers. When bicyclists race laps on an oval track each racer jockeys for second place rather then the lead position. The rider in second position benefits from the lead bike cutting through the wind resistance and prefers to draft comfortably until the finish line is in sight. Then at the very last moment, the second place racer slingshots past the lead rider, not at all unlike the action of your left palm in Twist and Strike. It's amazing to watch these racers in action, and amazing as well to feel how this unraveling action can enhance your Twist and Strike.

So far I've talked about waves, undertow, whale's fins, spear throwers, train wheel assemblies and bicycle racers. Nature and technology, always striving to be the best they can possibly be. In nature the "best" have evolutionary advantages. In technology the "best" gets market share. When you practice T'ai Chi you can always look at nature and technology to observe how and why the best is the best. No matter where you turn there's always a lesson to be had to improve your understanding of T'ai Chi. Conversely, the same lessons applied to your T'ai Chi can foster a richer experience and a greater appreciation of the world around you.

Notes

1. Wolinsky & Fitzgerald. *Journal of Gerontology*, 1994, p. 49.

2. *Journal of American Geriatrics*, 1996, vol. 44. See also, *Journal of the American Medical Association*, 1995, vol. 273.

3. B. Krolner. *Vertebral Bone Loss., Clinical Science 64,* 1983, quoted in *Better Bones, Better Bodies.* Susan Brown. 1996.

4. Susan Brown. *Better Bones, Better Bodies.* 1996.

5. Howard Gardner. *Frames of Mind.* 1993.

Ten Classical Principles of T'ai Chi Ch'uan:

1. Keep the top of the head (Bai Hui) light as if being held up, from above, by a string.
2. Let the focus and attention of the eyes direct your Ch'i, and be guided by the waist so as to remain congruent with the rest of the body.
3. Keep the chest and back slightly rounded (the chest concave, the back convex).
4. Relax the shoulders and allow the elbows to sink down to stay connected with the tailbone and the earth. Relax the wrist while the fingers elongate from within.
5. Sink your Ch'i into the lower abdomen (Dantien) and fill the kidneys.
6. Relax the perineum to sink the waist and tailbone down to the earth.
7. Curl the coccyx gently under to elongate the spine.
8. Keep the knees from extending forward beyond the toes.
9. Keep the knees from collapsing inward or outward.
10. Sink your energy to the earth, connecting through the Bubbling Well point.

Additional Principles:

1. Develop your ability to maintain your vertical centerline as an axis from the Bai Hui downwards through the perineum.

2. Develop your ability to always move fluidly from your center.

3. Maintain your root so that you do not bounce up.

4. Allow your spirit and intention to manifest within each movement.

5. Develop your Ting Jing skill in order to listen and perceive what needs to be perceived.

6. Always strive to integrate the different parts of your body, as well as the different parts of your self.

7. Always attend to strengthening the weakest part.

8. Breathe naturally.

9. Like water, seek the most natural path. Employ the least amount of force necessary for any given action.

10. When issuing force forward, root down to the back and draw in the front. When receiving force from the front, root to the front and ground down to the back.

11. Remember that both life and T'ai Chi are temporary gifts. Celebrate them accordingly.

Recommended Reading

Better Bones, Better Bodies, Brown, Keats Pub. Excellent book providing a refreshing and comprehensive approach to bone health for men and women.

Awaken Healing Energy Through the Tao, Chia. Aurora Press. Excellent primer on Taoist energy meditation. Step by step instruction on how to practice the Microcosmic Orbit.

Iron Shirt Ch'i Kung, Chia. Healing Tao Press. Clear and concise text on Taoist approach to energy and body structure via stationary postures.

Taoist Secrets of Love, Chia & Winn. *Healing Love Through the Tao*, Chia. Both Healing Tao Press. Both men's and women's versions, respectively, detailing Taoist approach to cultivation and management of sexual energy.

The Way of Qigong, Cohen. Ballantine Books. Seminal text, to date, addressing the myriad intricacies of this broad subject. Recommended!

The Moral Intelligence of Children. Coles, Plume. Deals nicely with a long ignored social and personal aspect of growth and development.

Encounters With Qi. Eisenberg M.D., David. West meets East in a timely validation of Chinese energy medicine.

Frames of Mind, Gardner, Challenges the old idea that intelligence is uni-dimensional. Gardner proposes seven distinct forms of intelligence.

Emotional Intelligence. Goleman. Bantam Books.

Embrace Tiger, Return to Mountain, Huang. Real People Press. Published back in 1973, now almost a cult book. This was the text that propelled T'ai Chi into the new-age awareness, promulgating its recognition as a mind/body discipline.

Full Catastrophe Living, Kabot-Zinn, Delta. Wonderful book by a pioneer in the field of blending eastern and western mind/body approaches for the purposes of pain management and personal wholeness.

Movements of Magic, Klein, Newcastle Pub. One of the few other books to explore T'ai Chi's efficacy as a mind/body discipline.

The Ten Essential Principles of T'ai Chi Ch'uan, Olsen, Dragon Door Pub. Pricey but delightful rendition of T'ai Chi's 10 Principles by the top student of T.T. Liang.

The Essence of Taiji Qigong, Yang. YMAA Publication Center For students who want to reach new levels of skill and ability in their existing forms.

Qigong for Health and Martial Arts, Yang. YMAA Publication Center A complete guide to Qigong training for all martial artists.

Tai Chi Theory & Martial Power, Yang. YMAA Publication Center. For advanced Yang style students. This book focuses on the martial aspect of Tai Chi Chuan, focusing on Jing training and the application of Chi in the Tai Chi form. It is a valuable reference book for Tai Chi practitioners.

T'AI CHI Magazine. PO 39938, LA, Ca, 90039. 1-800-888-9119.

Taijiquan Journal. PO 80538, Minneapolis, MN. 55408. (www.taijiquanjournal.com)

References

Brown, Susan E., Ph.D. (1996). *Better Bones, Better Body*, Keats Pub.

Chia, Mantak. (1983). *Awaken Healing Energy Through the Tao*, Aurora.

Chia, Mantak, (1986). *Iron Shirt Ch'i Kung*. Healing Tao Press. (HT Press).

Chia, Mantak & Maneewan. (1986). *Healing Love Through the Tao*. HT Press.

Chia, Mantak & Winn Michael. (1984). *Taoist Secrets of Love*. HT Press.

Chia, Mantak. (1985). *Taoist Ways to Transform Stress Into Vitality*. HT Press.

Chia, Mantak. (1989). *Fusion of the Five Elements*. HT Press.

Cohen, Ken. (1997). *The Way of Qigong*. Ballantine Books.

Frank, Douglas (1995). *Low Back Pain*. Blue Poppy Press

Gardner, Howard (1993). *Frames of Mind*. Basic. Basic books.

Gleick, James. (1988). *Chaos, Making a New Science*. Penguin USA.

Goleman, Daniel. (1994), *Emotional Intelligence*. Bantam

Huang, Al Chung-liang. (1973). *Embrace Tiger, Return to Mountain*. Real People Press.

Journal of American Geriatrics, 1996, vol. 44.

Journal of the American Medical Association, 1995, vol, 273.

Kabat- Zinn, Jon Ph.D. (1990). *Full Catastrophe Living*. Delta

Kapchuck, Ted. (1983). *The Web That Has No Weaver. Congdon & Weed.*

Klein, Bob (1983). *Movements of Magic*. Newcastle Books.

Krolner, B., and B. Toft. *Vertebral Bone Loss, An Unneeded Side Effect of Therapeutic Bed Rest*. Clin. Science 64 (1983).

Olsen, Stuart-Alve (1993). *The Ten Essential Principles of T'ai Chi Ch'uan*. Dragon Door Pub.

Master T.T. Liang. (1974). *T'ai Chi Ch'uan for Health and Self-defense*. Vintage Books.

Mitchell, Stephen. (1988). *Tao Te Ching*. Harper Perennial

Scott. W. Norman. (1996). *Scott's Knee Book*. Fireside

Selye, Hans. (1974). *Stress Without Distress*. Signet

Sky, Michael (1989). *Dancing With the Fire*. Bear & Co.

Vithoulkas, George. (1980). *The Science of Homeopathy*. Grove Weidenfeld

Wolinsky & Fitzgerald, 1994, 49, *Journal of Gerontology*.

Glossary of Terms

10,000 Things

Lao Tzu's (Lao Tse) reference in his Tao Te Ching to all things under Heaven that ever were, are, or shall be.

Asanas

Exercise postures common to (Hatha) yoga

Bai Hui (GV)-20)

The Bai Hui is located at the crown and may be found by tracing a line upwards from the tips of both ears to intersect at the sagittal sutures, which are formed by the joining of the fontanels (the spaces between the uncompleted angles of the parietal bones et al. of a fetal or young skull). The etymological derivation of "fontanel", is "little fountain"... a reference wholly compatible with the Taoist/TCM designation for this point.

Body/Mind

Throughout this book the reader will note my stubborn insistence on the use of the term "body/mind". On occasion, I address particular issues according to the manner in which they are more commonly regarded, as being more in the realm of the Body or of the Mind. Nevertheless, I believe the term body/mind accurately reflects the integrative approach of T'ai Chi at its best. In truth the Body, except possibly under rare and extreme medical circumstances, never exists in absence of the Mind. Nor does the Mind, except perhaps in rare esoteric circumstances, exist separate from the Body. I have never been able to delineate satisfactorily between the two.

Bubbling Well (Yung Chuan, K-1)

This first point on the Kidney meridian, at the bottom of each foot, is useful for rooting physically and energetically in T'ai Chi. You may locate this point by scrunching your bare foot and finding the center of the crease just behind the ball of the foot.

Ch'i (Qi)

Most simply and accurately described as life force energy. For the purposes of this book one may regard Ch'i as that energy which animates us as living beings. See chapter on Ch'i for a more detailed analysis.

Ch'i Kung (Qigong)

This is a term used to describe practices that combine the attention and intention of the mind with a conscious and deliberate attention to breath and/or movement. Use of this term is generally confined to a rather wide range of exercises adjunct to Chinese Kung Fu, T'ai Chi, or other internal art forms. Different Ch'i Kung practices can be categorized as simple, formulaic, or medical.

CNS

Central Nervous System

Coccyx (GV-1)

For the purposes of T'ai Chi, more accurately referred to as the sacral-coccygeal area, or simply the tailbone. The ability to articulate the tailbone as distinct from the ilium in which it is housed, is instrumental in properly connecting the upper and lower portions of the body. If this articulation is not cultivated fairly early in life, the coccyx, and its "housing", can fuse into an inseparable unit, as can sometimes be seen in students who undertake their study of T'ai Chi beyond middle age.

Dantien (Dondeen, CV-8)

The body's physical and energetic center, the Dantien can be experienced just behind and below the navel. It is a place where we receive nourishment and Ch'i pre-natally and remains a place where Ch'i can be safely stored and cultivated throughout our lives. (This actually is the lowest of the three dantiens, the other two being located at the Heart Center and the Third Eye.)

Empiricism

A philosophy that ascribes credibility to that which is perceived subjectively by the senses, versus only that which can be quantified objectively through logic or measurement.

Fa Jing

Term used to describe the execution of a move in T'ai Chi that is explosive and accompanied by a release of Ch'i energy.

Fascia

A membranous form of connective tissue that sheaths and supports the body's muscles and organs.

Homeopathy

Homeopathy is a non-traditional medical system, rooted in 17th century Germany, and promulgated on the theory of likes being used to cure likes, versus the anti's so prominent in traditional Western allopathic medicine.

Hui Yin (Perineum, CO-1)

Anatomically Western medicine regards this point as the small area between the anus and the genitals. In Chinese energy practices the area may be regarded as having a somewhat larger scope, from the coccyx forward to the genitals. The "Gate of Life and Death", as the perineum is known metaphorically, is significant because of its proximity to the body's many energy channels passing though the urogenital area. When properly aligned with the Bai Hui these two points serve in T'ai Chi to denote a centerline somewhat analogous to the axis of a revolving door.

I-Ching

Ancient and highly revered Chinese book of divination.

Iatrogenic

Induced unintentionally by one's doctor or medical environment, as in unintended 'side-effect', or an illness acquired as a result of hospitalization.

Internal Arts

Within the context of Chinese martial arts this term is generally understood to include T'ai Chi Ch'uan (Taijiquan), Pa-Kua Chang (Baguazhang), and Hsing I Chuan (Xingyiquan). A fourth, hybrid system, Liu He Ba Fa, is said to encompass the distinguishing characteristics of the first three systems. Various Ch'i Kung (Qigong) practices and meditation disciplines can also be included under this umbrella.

Jing

This is the term used in TCM to describe procreative, or sexual, energy. This energy is stored in the kidneys and is understood to govern the bones, as well as the reproductive function.

Kirlian photography

A photographic process developed in the 1970's which records the aura-like electrical discharge emanating from living objects.

Lao Kung (PC-6)

This point is located at the center of each palm. It is often the place where T'ai Chi practitioners first experience a conscious or tangible encounter with Ch'i energy.

Microcosmic Orbit

(a.k.a. Small Heavenly Circle, Wheel of the Law) The Microcosmic Orbit denotes a pattern and a process of moving Ch'i energy through the body in a completed circuit via the Functional (CV) and Governing vessels, two of the body's eight special channels.

Perineum

see Hui Yin

Proprioceptors

Sensory nerve endings, commonly found in muscles, tendons, joints, and the inner ear, that detect the motion or position of the body or a limb by responding to stimuli within the organism thus enabling balance and spatial orientation.

Qua (Kwa)

The Qua is a general term used to describe the loin/groin area, but may be specifically understood as a reference to the inguinal crease, which runs externally from approximately the forward crest of the ilium downwards and inwards to the pubic bone.

Rationalism

A theory first posited by Parmenides in ancient Greece, that endorses pure logic, versus intuition or empiricism, based on a presumed inherent unreliability of the senses to perceive reality objectively.

Tao

Universe, Heaven, all that was, is, and shall be. What came to be after there was nothing and will continue to be when all else is gone. The Tao is understood to be a self-regulating harmonic force.

Ting Jing (listening skill)

Ting Jing denotes one's ability to listen, or more accurately, perceive, via the sense of touch, where an opponent's energy is, or even what his intentions may be, simultaneous, or even prior, to their being manifested as an action. To avoid confusing internal arts neophytes and keep things simple I have opted to employ this one term broadly as an umbrella concept to encompass a range of related intrinsic T'ai Chi qualities including: Tung Jing—interpreting skill, Tsou Jing—receiving skill, Hua Jing—neutralizing skill, Yin Jing—enticing skill, et al.

TCM

Traditional Chinese Medicine

Thoracic Diaphragm

A band of muscular and connective tissue dividing the thoracic and abdominal cavities. Its contraction is what opens the lungs and causes breath to be drawn in. In many people the thoracic diaphragm becomes chronically engaged, thus contributing to constricted breathing patterns.

Wa

Japanese term denoting peaceful serenity

Wei Ch'i

Wei Ch'i is the body's first line of defense against illness and injury. Certain Ch'i Kung practices, such as Iron Shirt Ch'i Kung, are specifically intended to build this function to protect the body. In olden times, martial arts students were often required to practice such disciplines in order to endure the rigors of combat training. When strong the Wei Ch'i function acts like a bubble pack to mitigate the effects of shocking or jarring blows. A strong Wei Ch'i function also bolsters the body's immune system against what are known in Chinese medicine as "air" diseases, i.e. colds, flu, airborne contagions, etc.

Yi (ee)

A quality of the mind achieved by combining spirit with clear intention and focused attention.

Yin & Yang

These two forces represent polar opposites and exist as relative and necessary complements. Yin is regarded as feminine, dark, receiving, yielding, etc. Yang is masculine, light, issuing, and solid. Neither is absolute, and either in extreme ultimately begets its opposite.

Yuan Ch'i

Prenatal ch'i, Pre-birth, or Original Ch'i

About the Author

Sifu John Loupos began his study of martial arts in 1966 at the age of 13. At the age of 15, due to serendipitous circumstances, John inherited a school of his own and has been teaching martial arts ever since. Today John has a martial arts background spanning Okinawin Karate, Japanese Aikido, Filipino Arnis, and several Chinese Kung Fu systems including Bak Sil Lum, Choy Lay Fut, and Praying Mantis, plus Yang style T'ai Chi Ch'uan, Liu He Ba Fa, and Ba Gua Chang. John also practices and teaches Ch'i Kung and energy oriented meditation disciplines. He 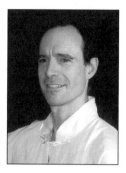 holds a B.A. in Psychology and is trained in Classical Homeopathy. His first book, *Tales & Strategies From the Jade Forest & Beyond*, addressed the issue of martial arts philosophy and morality for children.

John specializes in T'ai Chi Ch'uan as an inter- and intra-personal communication modality, and enjoys traveling to conduct seminars for educational and corporate entities as well as other schools. He currently lives at the shore in Hull, Massachusetts and busies himself with writing and teaching at his main school, Jade Forest Kung Fu/ T'ai Chi/ Internal Arts in Cohasset, Massachusetts plus two branch facilities.

The author welcomes comments and questions from readers. Please submit correspondence via the Jade Forest Kung Fu/T'ai Chi web site at www.jfkungfu.com or e-mail directly to jadeforest@attbi.com. Correspondance may also be submitted c/o the Publisher.

Index

BOOKS & VIDEOS FROM YMAA

YMAA Publication Center Books

YMAA Publication Center Videotapes

YMAA PUBLICATION CENTER 楊氏東方文化出版中心

4354 Washington Street Roslindale, MA 02131

1-800-669-8892 • ymaa@aol.com • www.ymaa.com